Civil Commitment in the Treatment of Eating Disorders

Civil Commitment in the Treatment of Eating Disorders presents a comprehensive view on the use of involuntary hospitalization in the treatment of patients with anorexia and other eating disorders. This volume synthesizes the existing empirical data and ethical perspectives surrounding this sometimes-controversial approach to treatment in order to establish a balanced, compassionate understanding of current research and patient experiences. Particular attention is paid to the use and misuse of persuasion and coercion in civil commitment and to when these concepts are applicable. This accessible new volume prepares treatment providers to understand the role of civil commitment in their treatment practices and in patients' recovery.

Wayne A. Bowers, PhD, ABPP, FAED, is clinical professor of psychiatry at the University of Iowa. He is a fellow in the Academy of Eating Disorders, as well as a founding fellow and certified CBT trainer and consultant in the Academy of Cognitive Therapy.

Civil Commitment in the Treatment of Eating Disorders

Practical and Ethical Considerations

Wayne A. Bowers

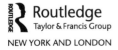

NEW YORK AND LONDON

First published 2018
by Routledge
711 Third Avenue, New York, NY 10017

and by Routledge
2 Park Square, Milton Park, Abingdon, Oxon, OX14 4RN

Routledge is an imprint of the Taylor & Francis Group, an informa business

© 2018 Taylor & Francis

The right of Wayne A. Bowers to be identified as author of this work
has been asserted by him in accordance with sections 77 and 78 of
the Copyright, Designs and Patents Act 1988.

All rights reserved. No part of this book may be reprinted or
reproduced or utilised in any form or by any electronic, mechanical,
or other means, now known or hereafter invented, including
photocopying and recording, or in any information storage or
retrieval system, without permission in writing from the publishers.

Trademark notice: Product or corporate names may be trademarks
or registered trademarks, and are used only for identification and
explanation without intent to infringe.

Library of Congress Cataloging-in-Publication Data
Names: Bowers, Wayne A., author.
Title: Civil commitment in the treatment of eating disorders :
    practical and ethical considerations / Wayne A. Bowers.
Description: New York, NY : Routledge, 2018. | Includes
    bibliographical references and index.
Identifiers: LCCN 2018003442 (print) | LCCN 2018004323
    (ebook) | ISBN 9781315457178 (eBook) |
    ISBN 9781138209435 (hardback) | ISBN 9781138209442 (pbk.) |
    ISBN 9781315457178 (ebk.)
Subjects: | MESH: Feeding and Eating Disorders—therapy |
    Commitment of Mentally Ill
Classification: LCC RC552.E18 (ebook) | LCC RC552.E18 (print) |
    NLM WM 175 | DDC 616.85/260651—dc23
LC record available at https://lccn.loc.gov/2018003442

ISBN: 978-1-138-20943-5 (hbk)
ISBN: 978-1-138-20944-2 (pbk)
ISBN: 978-1-315-45717-8 (ebk)

Typeset in Bembo
by Apex CoVantage, LLC

This book is dedicated to all the patients who have allowed me to help them make changes in their lives. They are unaware of how much they have taught me about their suffering and about life. For that I am forever grateful.

I want to acknowledge the love and support of my parents who encouraged me to be myself and to pursue what was important. They did not live to see this success. Also, I have no real words to offer those who have supported me for that past twenty years while I explored my personal and professional world. I want to express my undying appreciation and love for Marinan, Meghan, Lauren, Myca, Mielle, Christopher, Scott, and Kevin. Lastly, I am profoundly thankful to Georgia, whose love and compassion has kept me safe, on task, and makes my world a happier place.

Contents

Acknowledgments ix

Chapter 1   Basics of Eating Disorders   1

Chapter 2   History of Civil Commitment   19

Chapter 3   Civil Commitment and Eating Disorders   40

Chapter 4   Ethical Considerations   59

Chapter 5   Psychiatric Advanced Directives   77

Chapter 6   Compassionate Use of Civil Commitment   99

Chapter 7   Summary and Recommendations   111

Index 138

Acknowledgments

I would like to acknowledge those who have played a role in my development as a professional and a person. Professionally, I am grateful to the Center for Cognitive Therapy who gave me the opportunity to recognize and grow my therapy skills. Specifically, I want to thank Dr. Aaron Beck who gave me a chance to learn from a master therapist. I want to thank Dr. Brian Shaw who helped me appreciate the importance both comprehending and engaging in research. Equally important are the opportunities that were given me by the Department of Psychiatry at the University of Iowa. It was in this environment that I was able to develop practical aspects of treating individuals suffering from an eating disorder.

I want to thank Scott Temple, professional colleague, confidant, and long-time friend who has helped shape my understanding of cognitive therapy but more importantly the overall work of a psychotherapist. I am thankful to the warm acceptance of Craig Johnson and Joel Yager who helped me establish a position within the professional world working with eating disorders. Together, they encouraged me to bring my perspective to the field.

I am extremely grateful to Arnold Andersen who trusted me to be a professional colleague and friend while sharing his encyclopedic knowledge of individuals suffering from an eating disorder. Our work as a co-authors, discussions about treatment, and openness to new ideas with eating disorders offered opportunities to grow professionally. Finally, I want to thank each individual patient with an eating disorder who I have worked with over the past 40 years. They have taught me humility, patience, and an awareness regarding their struggle to change. Each one has made me a better professional but more importantly a better person.

1

Basics of Eating Disorders

Anorexia Nervosa

Eating disorders, primarily anorexia nervosa (AN) have been described in the literature for over 300 years (Bemporad, 1996). The *Diagnostic and Statistical Manual, Fifth Edition* (APA, 2013) identifies eight different eating disorders, with anorexia nervosa and bulimia nervosa being the most familiar. For purposes of this book I will focus on these two when looking at involuntary treatment and its ethical importance. Anorexia nervosa is diagnosed when an individual engages in deliberate self-induced weight loss, displays persistent restricted food intake, and has an intense fear of weight gain and/or of becoming fat. The disorder is associated with persistent and intrusive overvalued ideas regarding weight and shape, and an intense body image distortion. Symptoms can include restricted dietary choice, excessive exercise, self-induced vomiting, and purging by the use of appetite suppressants and diuretics. The disorder generally begins in adolescents or young adulthood and primarily affects women, but males can also suffer from the disorder (APA, 2013).

The first formal description of anorexia as a medical condition occurred in 1686 when Richard Morton (Bemporad, 1996), an

English physician, described a 20-year-old patient who was "a skeleton clad with skin" and wasting away (Gordon, 2000). In 1860 Louis-Victor Marce, a French psychiatrist, also described a patient who had symptoms similar to anorexia, hypothesizing a psychiatric origin (Silverman, 1997). Treatment recommendations included removing the patient from the family setting, force-feeding the individual if needed, and stopping all exercise (Garner & Garfinkel, 1994). Charles Lasegue, another French psychiatrist, observed a strong family component but characterized the problem as psychosocial in nature. A stressful home environment or family actions that suffocated the individual's emotional life were hypothesized as contributing to the development of the disorder (Kaufman & Heiman, 1964). However, Lasegue did not recommend a specific approach to treatment (Garner & Garfinkel, 1997). Careful observation and the use of the physician's authority could create change. Additionally, it was suggested that the patient be isolated from their family and only have visitors when there had been progress in treatment (Garner & Garfinkel, 1997).

In 1873 Sir William Gull coined the term "anorexia nervosa" meaning loss of appetite. He characterized the disease as a mental state rather than a biological disorder and advocated that patients be treated as rational rather than insane (Garner & Garfinkel, 1994). Treatment was based on rest, massage, consistent small meals to forced feeding, isolation from family, and surrounding the person with individuals who have moral control. Meals were to be presented to the patient by a nurse who interacted in a firm but compassionate and kind manner. Both Gull and Lasegue implied that this disorder was specific to women. However, by the turn of the century more physicians were reporting the disorder and suggested that the disorder could also be found among males (Brumberg, 2000, Hepworth, 1999). The writings of Gull and Lasegue are considered the foundation of understanding anorexia nervosa and their descriptions of the disorder remain almost identical to our understanding of the modern concept of AN. Following the appearance of their pioneer papers, anorexia nervosa became, by the turn of the century, a more recognizable disorder with the beginnings of subtyping based on food restriction or purging (Garner & Garfinkel, 1997).

Bulimia Nervosa

Bulimia nervosa (BN) is characterized by eating a large amount of food in a short period of time in which an individual feels completely out of control. Excessive preoccupation with control of body weight leads to a pattern of overeating generally followed by compensatory behavior designed to reverse the caloric intake and potential weight gain. Purging behavior includes self-induced vomiting, use of laxatives, diuretics, fasting, and excessive exercise. Bulimia nervosa shares many psychological characteristics with anorexia nervosa, including an overconcern with body shape and weight. A history of anorexia nervosa may be present with the interval ranging from a few months to several years (APA, 2013).

Bulimia nervosa was a rare disorder prior to the 20th century with few references to its existence. Pierre Janet, a French psychologist, described a patient in 1903 with anorexia nervosa who displayed secret compulsive eating behaviors (Gordon, 2000). The behaviors of this patient (episodic overeating, compensatory vomiting, fasting and/or laxative use, and a dread of getting fat) were consistent with the basic diagnostic criteria for bulimia nervosa. Mosche Wulff, a German psychoanalyst, also published a case study in 1932 of a patient using bingeing and purging to remain thin (DiNocola, 1990). In 1945 Ludwig Binswanger, a Swiss psychiatrist, described a case of a female patient who displayed bingeing, purging, and abuse of laxatives to remain thin (DiNocola, 1990). Dr. Marlene Boskind-Lodahl (Boskind-Lodahl, 1976, Boskind-Lodahl & White, 1977, Boskind-Lodahl & White 1978) described her work with a series of 138 women that she treated for an eating disorder. Her publication in 1976 highlighted the problem of eating disorders on college campuses and coined the term "bulimarexia" (Gordon, 2000).

Dr. Gerald Russell published the first formal paper on bulimia nervosa in 1979, characterizing it as a distinct variant of anorexia (Russell, 1979). Prominent symptoms of bulimia included bingeing, purging, and preoccupation with body shape and weight. Fear of fatness was similar to anorexia nervosa but the compensatory mechanisms relied primarily on vomiting, use of laxatives, diuretics, diet pills, fasting, and excessive exercise. According to Dr. Russell, anorexia and bulimia nervosa are developmental disorders that share similar features such as over valuation of weight and shape, a fear of becoming fat, and body image concerns (Vogler, 1993).

Prevalence, Onset, and Course of Eating Disorders

Eating disorders are relatively rare and are more commonly seen in women. Only about 10% of patients diagnosed with anorexia or bulimia are male, but there is a suggestion that these data are likely an underestimate of the prevalence of males who are less likely to admit to having eating problems and less likely to seek help compared to women (APA, 2013). Lifetime prevalence statistics suggest that about 0.5% of women and 0.05% of men will meet criteria for anorexia during their lifetimes. Between 2% and 3% of women and 0.02% to 0.03% of men will meet the criteria for bulimia nervosa during their lifetimes (Westmoreland & Mehler, 2016). The average age of onset for anorexia displays bimodal peaks between ages 13–14 and 17–18 for females, while males are somewhat older with onset between ages 18 and 19 (APA, 2013). Despite these important differences in frequency and onset age, there is consensus within the scientific literature that eating disorders in the male population are otherwise very similar in nature to those in the female population (APA, 2013).

The course and outcome of eating disorders vary significantly across different people. Experts believe that approximately 75%–80% who suffer from an eating disorder will have improved from their disorder in 15 years (Arcelus, Mitchell, Wales, & Nielsen, 2011). A small proportion of individuals with this disorder suffer for their entire lives. However, between 6% and 20% of eating disordered individuals will die as a result of their disease, and anorexia has the highest mortality rate of all psychiatric illnesses (Arcelus et al., 2011).

Psychological Complications

In general, people who develop an eating disorder share intense concerns about weight and shape that can have a profound effect on self-esteem. Individuals diagnosed with an eating disorder feel badly about their body image and are not able to physically or psychological see themselves as others perceive them (Fairburn 2003, 2008). These body image concerns and body image distortions contribute to an overall personal sense of dysphoria and interpersonal ineffectiveness. A common predicament of too many individuals with an eating disorder is sensitivity to social acceptance, perfectionism, and a tendency to establish unrealistically high standards. Experiencing any or all of these concerns can lead to frustration and self-criticism about their self-worth and overall value in the world (Fairburn, 2003, 2008). The development of an eating disorder may be a compensatory strategy to cope with these perceived failures, which in turn lead to working harder to achieve their impossible goals. This emotional distress in turn leads to further neglect of their physical and psychological condition, leading to disruption of their life and potential death (Touyz & Hay, 2015). According to a transdiagnostic model, all eating disorders share the same set of dysfunctional beliefs (Fairburn, 2003, 2008). These beliefs, often referred to as core psychopathology include negative beliefs about self-worth, a desire for control and over-evaluation of body weight and appearance, and their control (Fairburn, 2003).

Medical Complications

Eating disorders affect the thoughts, feelings, and behavior of an individual but also disrupt multiple physical aspects of the body, some of which can become life-threatening (Mehler & Andersen, 2017, Westmoreland, Krantz, & Mehler, 2016). Dieting, poor nutrition, purging and abuse of laxatives, among other things can set the stage for medical complications that can affect every organ system in the body. Starvation and chaotic eating can disrupt electrolytes leading to serious heart problems such as decreased size of the heart muscle, a disruption of blood pressure, bradycardia, and arrhythmias (Mehler & Andersen, 2017, Westmoreland et al., 2016). More specifically, low potassium can lead to diminished reflexes, fatigue, and potential cardiac abnormalities that may not resolve. Other consequences of restricted caloric intake or chaotic eating can include a feeling of weakness, confusion, poor concentration, seizures, and death (Mehler & Andersen, 2017, Westmoreland et al., 2016). Poor nutrition has been implicated in the development of anemia, anxiety, restlessness, or fainting for individuals who develop an eating disorder. A long-term nonreversible condition related to starvation is osteopenia, reflecting poor bone mineral density leading to premature weakness or brittleness in one's bones. Without intervention into this starvation-related problem, osteopenia becomes a precursor to osteoporosis (Mehler & Andersen, 2017, Westmoreland et al., 2016).

Binge eating and chronic vomiting contributes to dental problems such as caries and erosion of tooth enamel. It can also lead to a sensation of fullness, feeling bloated, gastric distress, and damage to the lining of the stomach. Tearing or rupturing of the esophagus and stomach can also occur due to the pressure of binge eating and vomiting, causing serious, life-threatening medical problems (Mehler & Andersen, 2017, Westmoreland et al., 2016). Gastroesophageal reflux disease, a potentially life-threatening condition, occurs when the contents of the stomach, including acid, back up into the esophagus causing inflammation and heartburn symptoms. Untreated, this can lead to Barrett's esophagus, which leads to precancerous changes in the esophagus (Mehler & Andersen, 2017, Westmoreland et al., 2016). Individuals with bulimia nervosa can experience lung aspiration (inhaling foreign matter, typically vomit, into the lungs), causing damage to lung tissue, pneumonia, shock, and/or respiratory disease. Other common medical complications of a poor diet include constipation, abdominal pain, bladder incontinence, and urinary tract infections. In a starved individual there is growth of long, downy hair on the face, arms, and body (called lanugo)—a sign that the body is attempting to stay warm (Mehler & Andersen, 2017, Westmoreland et al., 2016).

Other medical concerns include delayed or permanently stunted growth, severe dehydration which can lead to water retention (edema), and impaired kidney functioning. Also, a metabolic imbalance called alkalosis (an imbalance of pH levels in the blood and body fluids) causes symptoms ranging from slowed breathing to coma (Mehler & Andersen, 2017, Westmoreland et al., 2016).

Reduced fat intake contributes to skin elasticity, loss of hair, and brittle fingernails. The central nervous system can also be disrupted with enlarged lateral ventricles and cortical sulci which correlates with amount of weight loss. Also, gray matter can be reduced, which can persist even after weight restoration (Mehler & Andersen, 2017, Westmoreland et al., 2016).

High Risk of Mortality

As evident, eating disorders (primarily anorexia nervosa) can be very dangerous, even lethal, if not treated. Overall crude mortality rate is 3.9%, with the highest percentage in AN patients and the lowest percentage in BN patients (Arcelus et al., 2011, Fichter & Quadflieg, 2016). For BN there is significant improvement over the short term, with 50% recovered at 5-year follow-up, and 70% of individuals having improved in their symptoms after 10 years (Arcelus et al., 2011, Fichter & Quadflieg, 2016). However, a recent meta-analysis of BN found standard mortality rates to be mildly elevated (SMR = 1.93), considerably lower than for AN but, for BN, still significantly elevated as compared to the general population, suggesting the importance of adequate care. The SMR for AN was 5.35 and thus, more than five times higher than the mortality in the general population matched for age and sex (Arcelus et al., 2011, Fichter & Quadflieg, 2016).

As suggested, anorexia nervosa has one of the highest mortality rates of all mental disorders. The National Eating Disorders Association indicates that 5%–20% of those who have untreated anorexia nervosa will not survive the disorder (Theander, 1983). The annual death rate for females between 15 and 24 years old from anorexia is 12 times higher than the annual death rate for all other causes combined (Eckert, Halmi. Marchi, Grove, & Crosby, 1995). Although most studies report a death rate of less than 8%, several report a rate greater than 15%. Longer-term studies tend to show higher mortality rates (Steinhausen, 2002, Halmi, Brodland, & Rigas, 1975, Baran, Weltzin, & Kaye, 1995, Theander, 1983, 1992, Ratnasuriya, Eisler, Szmukler, & Russell, 1991). The most notable of these, a Scandinavian study conducted over 22 years, found an 18% mortality (Theander, 1983). Approximately 75% of deaths are from natural causes such as electrolyte disturbance, circulatory collapse, cachexia, and organ failure, with suicide also a significant contributor (Theander, 1983). Fully two-thirds of all anorexia nervosa nonnatural deaths were attributable to suicide, with rates estimated between 1% and 5% (Steinhausen, 2002, Halmi et al., 1975, Baran et al., 1995, Theander, 1983, 1992, Ratnasuriya et al., 1991). For those who receive treatment, the mortality rate is far lower—approximately 2%–3% of these people will die from this disorder, but it is still life-threatening.

Impaired Judgment

The starvation and chaotic eating in these disorders can lead to concerns about the cognitive functioning for these individuals. Two areas that have been highlighted as problems are executive functioning and poor set-shifting. This is especially troublesome with anorexia nervosa. These cognitive deficits have been associated with a poor long-term outcome, a longer duration of illness, low self-esteem and increased depression and anxiety, and more severe eating disorder behavior (Hirst et al., 2017, Harper, Brodrick, Van Enkevort, & McAdams, 2017). Additionally, cognitive disturbances may be a factor that reduces an individual's ability to understand (insight) the extent or the severity of their disorder, thereby maintaining the illness (Hirst et al., 2017, Harper et al., 2017). This can then affect treatment engagement and lead to treatment refusal. Resistance to treatment can contribute to poorer health with the ultimate negative outcome of death.

Treatment Refusal

As can be seen, the consequences of an eating disorder can impair multiple aspects of the individual's ability to adequately understand the extent of the disorder. As such, when approached by others who want to help to change the individual's behavior, there is a high likelihood of refusal (Carney, Tait, & Touyz, 2007, Charland, 2013, Goldner, Birmingham, & Smye, 1997, Goldner, McKenzie, & Kline, 1991, Ryan & Callaghan, 2014, Tan & Richards, 2015, Tan, Hope, Stewart, & Fitzpatrick, 2006, 2008).

Medical complications (starvation), overvalued beliefs (I must be thin to be special), and distorted body image (seeing oneself as fat when not), singly or in combination, can make it very difficult to assist the individual to change. Refusal of treatment is often explained rationally by the individual as something they can alter anytime they want. But it can also take the form of a more adversarial stance by the individual who wishes to be left alone and who insists that nothing is wrong (Carney et al., 2007, Charland, 2013, Goldner et al., 1997, Goldner et al., 1991, Ryan & Callaghan, 2014, Tan & Richards, 2015, Tan et al., 2008). These beliefs make it hard to help the individual understand the physical, social, and psychological consequences of their disorder, in turn leading to short-term medical problems (poor digestive health) or long-term difficulties such as irreversible cardiac problems, poor bone health, and in a small number of individuals, death. These negative outcomes can also lead caring friends, family, and health care professionals to increase pressure on the affected individual to change, which can be met with more resistance. Empirical data indicate that the longer the individual goes untreated, the worse the long-term outcome. The perceived importance of the disorder to the affected individual places other aspects of their life (work, school, social life) at such a low importance they limit their chances for success in school, interpersonal, and family relationships (Carney et al., 2007, Charland, 2013, Goldner et al., 1997, Goldner et al., 1991, Ryan & Callaghan,2014, Tan & Richards, 2015, Tan et al., 2008).

Some individuals feel helpless to effect change and consider having others step in to help return them to their previous level of physical and psychological health. However, this request can be undermined by the belief that the disorder is a part of their "person" and changing would alter their personal essence (Tan et al., 2008). However, the absence of treatment can lead to long-term interference of the individual's world, depriving them of the likelihood of a successful life. Treatment refusal must therefore be addressed in a manner that respects the individual while helping them get well. Safeguarding the health and well-being of the individual becomes paramount. However, the means to restore health can be contentious, and working in the "best interest" of the individual is not always agreed upon. Legitimate methods to accomplish a return to health may include persuasive and coercive means (Tan et al., 2008). Without treatment a severe and enduring type of disorder can develop (Carney, Tait, Richardson, & Touyz, 2008).

Severe and Enduring Eating Disorders

Severe and enduring aspects of eating disorders (primarily anorexia) are a poorly understood subgroup of patients with malignant, chronic anorexia nervosa (APA, 2006, Fedyszyn & Sullivan, 2007, Strober, 2006). Described under various names (severe and enduring eating disorder [SEED], severe and enduring-anorexia nervosa [SE-AN]), individuals with this subtype are basically similar. As described by several authors (Robinson, Kukucska, Guidetti, & Leavey, 2015, Touyz & Hay, 2015, Strober, 2006, Fedyszyn & Sullivan, 2007), treatment may have minimal impact on the persistent and unrelenting eating disorder symptoms which are so characteristic of those with severe and enduring eating disorder. As most information about this subgroup focuses on anorexia, I will use severe and enduring anorexia nervosa (SE-AN) to simplify the discussion.

As a subgroup there is no implication of clinical nihilism or giving up on the patient but rather a change in focus in how we interact. As noted, the high mortality rate and multiple medical complications for individuals with an eating disorder suggests that those with SE-AN have a reduced life expectancy, have more psychosocial disruption, and create a challenge for health care professionals (Munro et al., 2014, Dawson, Rhodes, & Touyz, 2014). With a reduced likelihood of change or recovery for this group, it is important to identify methods to keep these individuals engaged in treatment. New models are being described that focus on the needs of the whole person, their quality of life, and medical stability while reducing emphasis on weight gain and restoration (Munro et al., 2014, Dawson et al., 2014). Patients with SE-AN can no longer be ignored, for they have suffered for far too long, contending with an abysmal quality of life devoid of any hope of an effective treatment on the horizon (Munro et al., 2014, Dawson et al., 2014).

Those living with SE-AN want to be validated and to feel understood by their friends, family, and health care professionals (Munro et al., 2014, Dawson et al., 2014). Health care professionals and families struggle with how to help engage their loved ones in treatment looking for answers that include involuntary treatment and the ethics of palliative care. It is the use of civil commitment that families and caregivers find difficult to discuss and implement medically legal methods that have the potential to sustain life (Munro et al., 2014, Dawson et al., 2014).

Legal policy often cannot be avoided in the treatment of chronic patients, and most notably involves involuntary commitment, legal incompetency, and guardianship for patients below the age of majority.

When the behavior of these patients endangers their lives, they will usually be committable under grave disability standards (Goldner, McKenzie, & Kline, 1991, Goldner, 1989, Goldner, Birmingham, & Smye, 1997). There is a consensus that involuntary commitment should be used as an approach of last resort, when patients decline voluntary hospitalization and their physical safety is at risk. Civil commitment should probably also be limited to circumstances in which therapeutic gain is likely from hospitalization (APA, 2006). Safeguarding the individual can become paramount and coercion can be seen as legitimate instrument to restore health that is in the individual's best interest (Tan et al., 2003). Goldner (1989) offers a view of treatment refusal that suggests that clinicians may need to refuse treatment in exceptional cases as an "ultimatum" to provide a confrontation regarding the lack of collaboration in the treatment.

References

American Psychiatric Association. (2006). Treatment of patients with eating disorders (3rd ed.). *American Journal of Psychiatry*, 163(7 Suppl), 4–54.

American Psychiatric Association. (2013). *Diagnostic and statistical manual of mental disorders (DSM-5)*. Washington, DC: American Psychiatric Association.

Arcelus, J., Mitchell, A.J., Wales, J., & Nielsen, S. (2011). Mortality rates in patients with anorexia nervosa and other eating disorders: A meta-analysis of 36 studies. *Archives of General Psychiatry*, 68(7), 724–731.

Baran, S.A., Weltzin, T.E., & Kaye, W.H. (1995). Low discharge weight and outcome in anorexia nervosa. *American Journal of Psychiatry*, 152(7), 1070.

Bemporad, J.R. (1996). Self-starvation through the ages: Reflections on the pre-history of anorexia nervosa. *International Journal of Eating Disorders*, 19(3), 217–237.

Boskind-Lodahl, M. (1976). Cinderella's stepsisters: A feminist perspective on anorexia nervosa and bulimia. *Signs: Journal of Women in Culture and Society*, 2(2), 342–356.

Boskind-Lodahl, M., & White, W.C., Jr. (1978). The definition and treatment of bulimarexia in college women—A pilot study. *Journal of American College Health Association*, 27(2), 84–97.

Brumberg, J.J. (2000). *Fasting girls: The history of anorexia nervosa*. New York: Vintage Books.

Carney, T., Tait, D., Richardson, A., & Touyz, S. (2008). Why (and when) clinicians compel treatment of anorexia nervosa patients. *European Eating Disorders Review*, 16(3), 199–206.

Carney, T., Tait, D., & Touyz, S. (2007). Coercion is coercion? Reflections on trends in the use of compulsion in treating anorexia nervosa. *Australasian Psychiatry*, 15(5), 390–395.

Charland, L.C. (2013). Ethical and conceptual issues in eating disorders. *Current Opinion in Psychiatry*, 26(6), 562–565.

Dawson, L., Rhodes, P., & Touyz, S. (2014). "Doing the Impossible": The process of recovery from chronic anorexia nervosa. *Qualitative Health Research*, 24(4), 494–505.

DiNocola, V.F.C. (1990). Anorexia multiforms: Self starvation in historical and cultural context. *Transcultural Psychiatric Research Review*, 27, 165–196.

Eckert, E.D., Halmi, K.A., Marchi, P., Grove, W., & Crosby, R. (1995). Ten-year follow-up of anorexia nervosa: Clinical course and outcome. *Psychological Medicine*, 25(1), 143–156.

Fairburn, C.G. (2008). *Cognitive behavior therapy and eating disorder*. New York: Guilford Press.

Fedyszyn, I.E., & Sullivan, G.B. (2007). Ethical re-evaluation of contemporary treatments for anorexia nervosa: Is an aspirational stance possible in practice? *Australian Psychologist*, 42(3), 198–211.

Fichter, M.M., & Quadflieg, N. (2016). Mortality in eating disorders—results of a large prospective clinical longitudinal study. *International Journal of Eating Disorders*, 49(4), 391–401.

Garner, D.M., & Garfinkel, P.E. (Eds.). (1997). *Handbook of treatment for eating disorders*. New York: Guilford Press.

Goldner, E. (1989). Treatment refusal in anorexia nervosa. *International Journal of Eating Disorders*, 8(3), 297–306.

Goldner, E.M., Birmingham, C.L., & Smye, V. (1997). Addressing treatment refusal in anorexia nervosa: Clinical, ethical, and legal considerations. In D.M. Garner & P.E. Garfinkel (Eds.), *Handbook of Treatment for Eating Disorders*, 2, 450–461.

Goldner, E.M., McKenzie, J.M., & Kline, S.A. (1991). The ethics of forced feeding in anorexia nervosa. *CMAJ: Canadian Medical Association Journal*, 144(10), 1205.

Gordon, R.A. (2000). *Eating disorders: Anatomy of a social epidemic*. Malden, MA: Blackwell.

Halmi, K., Brodland, G., & Rigas, C. (1975). A follow-up study of 79 patients with anorexia nervosa: an evaluation of prognostic factors and diagnostic criteria. *Life History Review Psychopathology*, 4, 290–300.

Harper, J.A., Brodrick, B., Van Enkevort, E., & McAdams, C.J. (2017). Neuropsychological and cognitive correlates of recovery in anorexia nervosa. *European Eating Disorders Review*, 25(6), 491–500.

Hepworth, J. (1999). *The social construction of anorexia nervosa.* Thousand Oaks, CA: Sage.

Hirst, R.B., Beard, C.L., Colby, K.A., Quittner, Z., Mills, B., & Lavender, J.M. (2017). Anorexia nervosa and bulimia nervosa: A meta-analysis of executive functioning. *Neuroscience & Biobehavioral Reviews*, 83, 678–690.

Kaufman, R.M., & Heiman, M.E. (1964). *Evolution of psychosomatic concepts* (pp. 132–136). New York: International Universities Press. Gull W.W. Anorexia nervosa, reprinted in Kaufman, M.R., Herman, M., 1873.

Mehler, P.S., & Andersen, A.E. (2017). *Eating disorders: A guide to medical care and complications* (3rd ed.). Baltimore, MD: Johns Hopkins Press.

Munro, C., Thomson, V., Corr, J., Randell, L., Davies, J.E., Gittoes, C., . . . Freeman, C.P. (2014). A new service model for the treatment of severe anorexia nervosa in the community: The anorexia nervosa intensive treatment team. *Psychiatric Bulletin*, 38(5), 220–225.

Ratnasuriya, R.H., Eisler, I., Szmukler, G.I., & Russell, G.F.M. (1991). Anorexia nervosa: outcome and prognostic factors after 20 years. *British Journal of Psychiatry*, 158(4), 495–502.

Robinson, P.H., Kukucska, R., Guidetti, G., & Leavey, G. (2015). Severe and enduring anorexia nervosa (SEED-AN): A qualitative study of patients with 20+ years of anorexia nervosa. *European Eating Disorders Review*, 23(4), 318–326.

Russell, G. (1979). Bulimia nervosa: An ominous variant of anorexia nervosa. *Psychological Medicine*, 9, 429–448.

Ryan, C.J., & Callaghan, S. (2014). Treatment refusal in anorexia nervosa: The hardest of cases. Commentary on "Anorexia Nervosa: The Diagnosis: A Postmodern Ethics Contribution to the Bioethics Debate on Involuntary Treatment for Anorexia Nervosa" by Sacha Kendall. *Journal of Bioethical Inquiry*, 11(1), 43–45.

Silverman, J.A. (1997). Anorexia nervosa: Historical perspective on treatment. In D.M. Garner & P.E. Garfinkel (Eds.), *Handbook of treatment for eating disorders* (pp. 3–10). New York: Guilford Press.

Steinhausen, H.C. (2002). The outcome of anorexia nervosa in the 20th century. *American Journal of Psychiatry*, 159(8), 1284–1293.

Strober, M. (2006). Managing the chronic, treatment resistant patient with anorexia nervosa. *International Journal of Eating Disorders*, 36, 245–255.

Tan, J.O., Hope, T., Stewart, A., & Fitzpatrick, R. (2006). Competence to make treatment decisions in anorexia nervosa: Thinking processes and values. *Philosophy, Psychiatry, & Psychology: PPP*, 13(4), 267.

Tan, J.O., Hope, T., Stewart, A., & Fitzpatrick, R. (2008). Control and compulsory treatment in anorexia nervosa: The views of patients and parents. *International Journal of Law and Psychiatry*, 26(6), 627–645.

Tan, J., & Richards, L. (2015). Legal and ethical issues in the treatment of really sick patients with anorexia nervosa. In *Critical care for anorexia nervosa* (pp. 113–150). Berlin: Springer International.

Theander, S. (1983). Research on outcome and prognosis of anorexia nervosa and some results from a Swedish long-term study. *International Journal of Eating Disorders*, 2(4), 167–174.

Theander, S. (1992). Chronicity in anorexia nervosa: Results from the Swedish long-term study. In W. Herzog, H. Deter, & W. Vandereycken (Eds.), *The course of eating disorders* (pp. 214–227). Berlin: Springer.

Touyz, S., & Hay, P. (2015). Severe and enduring anorexia nervosa (SE-AN): In search of a new paradigm. *Journal of Eating Disorders*, 3(1), 26.

Vogler, R.J. (1993). *The medicalization of eating: Social control in an eating disorders clinic*. Greenwich, CT: Jai Press.

Westmoreland, P., Krantz, M.J., & Mehler, P.S. (2016). Medical complications of anorexia nervosa and bulimia. *American Journal of Medicine*, 129(1), 30–37.

Westmoreland, P., & Mehler, P.S. (2016). Caring for patients with severe and enduring eating disorders (SEED): Certification, harm reduction, palliative care, and the question of futility. *Journal of Psychiatric Practice*, 22(4), 313–320.

2

History of Civil Commitment

Introduction

Civil commitment or compulsory treatment for psychiatric disorders has been in existence for more than 150 years (Testa & West, 2010). How and when civil commitment has been implemented has evolved over the years to reflect the ideas of community, mental health professionals, and the law. The use of involuntary hospitalization has been argued as a critical first step in psychiatric care and has been seen as a mainstay to the initiation of psychiatric care (Testa & West, 2010). Patients whose incapacity to assist in their own treatment, denial of the illness, or refusal of treatment leads to life-threatening or life-impeding outcomes are often embroiled in civil commitment.

Balancing the treatment needs of the mentally ill with protection of personal freedom and civil liberty is one of the greatest challenges of civil commitment law. The first European institutions specifically for people with mental illness were established in 1403 in London, England, and in 1407 in Valencia, Spain. Unfortunately, Europeans increasingly isolated mentally ill people, often housing them with people who had physical handicaps, vagrants, and delinquents. Additionally, those considered insane were treated inhumanely, often chained to walls and kept in dungeons. Concern about the treatment of people with mental illness grew to the point that occasional reforms were instituted. After the French Revolution, French physician Philippe Pinel took over the Bicêtre Hospital and stopped the use of chains and shackles. He also removed patients from dungeons, provided sunny rooms, and allowed exercise.

In England in the 19th century, individuals with mental illness were often treated as subhuman and were housed in prisons. The authority of two justices of the peace could involuntarily detain an individual with mental illness. During the Victorian era there was a movement to provide more positive structure and compassionate care. Early asylums, although a step forward, were still patterned after penitentiaries. More humane hospital environments were eventually legislated into existence and included inspection of private and public hospitals with the intent of balancing the protection of society while protecting patients against abuse. At this time in history, civil commitment was usually instituted by a relative or other person supported by two medical doctors. Mental health legislation relied upon the family as protector of patients, but left patients unprotected from improper detention at the instigation of relatives. By the 1890s civil commitment was in the hands of a magistrate or county judge (Fennell & Goldstein, 2006, Jacobsen, 2012).

In the United States, prior to the Revolutionary War, mentally ill individuals who could not care for themselves and lacked family supervision or support were typically ignored or managed in jails or houses for the poor. Philadelphia created the first psychiatric hospital in 1752 and by the early decades of the 19th century a few small private and public facilities had developed across the states. Between 1817 and 1824, four privately funded asylums were established in the northeastern states of Connecticut, New York, Massachusetts, and Pennsylvania. Admissions were always involuntary, typically initiated by family or friends, and the length of stay was linked to ongoing private financial support. Hospital treatment was coerced, since it was presumed that mentally ill patients were too disabled to request (or refuse) care on their own behalf. These early commitment laws focused more on the need for treatment with the state acting in *parens patriae*, the traditional power to care for those incapable of caring for themselves (Anfang & Appelbaum, 2006, Appelbaum, 2006, Fennell & Goldstein, 2006).

In the early 20th century, "psychopathic hospitals" dedicated to caring for acute cases were developed in major cities in the hope that early intervention and treatment would have greater therapeutic impact. States developed special emergency commitment procedures that would bypass time-consuming judicial hearings, allowing physicians (and sometimes police) to hospitalize patients for brief periods of time without court review.

By the 1950s, care of all mental health problems was operating under a single legal framework. Also, tribunals were established to oversee the legality of civil commitment and its continuation. The tribunals consisted of a legally qualified president, a psychiatrically qualified medical member, and a third member with expertise in the operation of the mental health system. To be civilly committed, a patient had to be suffering from a mental disorder of a nature or degree warranting detention for assessment and/or treatment. When treatment was necessary, it had to be in the interest of the patient's health or safety or for the protection of others (Fennell & Goldstein, 2006, Jacobsen, 2012).

In 1951, the newly established National Institute of Mental Health (NIMH) issued the landmark "Draft Act Governing Hospitalization of the Mentally Ill," which proposed streamlining commitment procedures, including a certification process that was entirely in medical hands (Anfang & Appelbaum, 2006). The NIMH Draft Act proposed a modified version of the traditional "need for treatment" formula. To involuntarily hospitalize a person, there must be proof that the individual is in need of care or treatment in a mental hospital. Additionally, the individual must lack sufficient insight or capacity to make responsible decisions (Anfang & Appelbaum, 2006, Fennell & Goldstein, 2006).

Dangerousness as the sole ground for civil commitment was first adopted by the District of Columbia in 1964 and then by California. California's 1969 Lanterman-Petris-Short Act permitted civil commitment only for those who were imminently dangerous to themselves or to others, or who were so "gravely disabled" as to be unable to meet their minimal needs for survival (Anfang & Appelbaum, 2006). This approach to involuntary hospitalization quickly became the model for many U.S. states. Need for treatment was no longer a substantive factor for civil commitment. By the end of the 1970s, nearly every state had revised its commitment statutes to conform to the dangerousness criteria (www.treatmentadvoca cycenter.org/). Over the past 20 years several states have broadened the definition of "grave disability" for inpatient commitment to include the prospect of severe deterioration, disabling illness, or general inability to care for oneself (Anfang & Appelbaum, 2006, Testa & West, 2010).

In the United States, all 50 states have statutes regarding civil commitment for psychiatric disorders. However, those statutes vary from state to state. In eight states, the sole ground for civil commitment is dangerousness, which means an individual must demonstrate an immediate, physical danger to self or others before a court can intervene and order treatment. In the remaining 42 states, laws permit intervention based on additional criteria that is broader than dangerousness to self or others and is usually referred to as grave disability (Treatment Advocacy Center, 2013). Grave disability typically focuses on the person's inability to meet his or her basic survival needs. More specifically, gravely disabled means a condition in which a person, as a result of a mental disorder, is in danger of serious physical harm resulting from a failure to provide for his or her essential human needs such as food, clothing, or shelter. Conversely, even if there is a serious mental disorder, the individual can voluntarily request family, friends, or others to assist in meeting his/her needs. When family members, friends, or others are willing and able to help provide for the person's basic needs regarding food, clothing, or shelter and with this assistance the individual has the ability to survive safely without involuntary detention, then there is no grave disability. In essence, a person is not gravely disabled if family members or others are willing to help and if the person receiving this help can take care of his/her basic needs.

A third provision in which a court can intervene in a mental health crisis is called need for treatment. Need-for-treatment standards (which are found in 26 states) include qualification for care based on at least one of the following conditions: (1) the person's inability to provide for needed psychiatric care; (2) the person's inability to make an informed medical decision; and (3) the person's need for intervention to prevent further psychiatric or emotional deterioration (Treatment Advocacy Center, 2013). Though the extent of states' power to commit mentally ill persons on a "need-for-treatment" basis remains unclear, the U.S. Supreme Court will allow the states considerable leeway in defining mental illness, "danger to self or others," and "gravely disabled" (Treatment Advocacy Center, 2013).

Forty-six states permit the use of assisted outpatient treatment (AOT), also known as outpatient commitment or court-ordered outpatient treatment. Assisted outpatient treatment is court-ordered treatment (including medication) for individuals with symptoms of severe mental illness who meet strict legal criteria (e.g., they have a history of medication noncompliance). Studies and data from states using AOT have found that it is effective in reducing the incidents and duration of hospitalization, homelessness, arrests and incarcerations, victimization, violent episodes, and other consequences of nontreatment. AOT can increase treatment compliance and promotes long-term voluntary compliance (Treatment Advocacy Center, 2013). Typically, violation of the court-ordered conditions can result in the individual being hospitalized for further treatment (Geller, 2006, Honig & Stefan, 2005).

As can be seen, the evolution of modern civil commitment is a complex set of interactions among state legislatures, lay and professional interest groups, and the judicial system. Financial support from governments in the area of mental health, legislative changes at the state and federal levels, and increased emphasis on personal civil rights and liberties have all shaped how and when civil commitment is utilized (Anfang & Appelbaum, 2006, Appelbaum, 2006, Bloom, 2004). These factors have led to a decline in the acceptance of civil commitment as a vehicle to assist the emotionally troubled individual. However, with the concept of grave disability becoming more prominent in state statutes and more states enacting outpatient commitment statutes, civil commitment again appears to be a viable option. Unfortunately, balancing the desire to help the "gravely disabled" and fear of restricting the individual's personal liberty makes it hard to create a consistently fair, reasonable, and compassionate civil commitment law. By merging the experience in the United States with the experience and the experiments of other nations, we can create a uniform and empathetic view of civil commitment (Anfang & Appelbaum, 2006, Appelbaum, 2006, Bloom, 2004).

International Civil Commitment

Internationally, civil commitment laws range from very strict legislation to none at all. Many Western countries use similar language in their legislation when it comes to civil commitment but specifics vary by region or state. The European Union legally permits compulsory admission of the mentally ill only when a less restrictive environment might not be adequate or available. Compulsory admission is the intervention of last resort, or applied only in an acute crisis or state of emergency. Criteria for civil commitment in the European Union is categorized into three groups. A serious threat of harm to the self and/or to others ("dangerousness criterion") is an essential prerequisite for compulsory admission in Austria, Belgium, France, Germany, Luxembourg, and the Netherlands. Along with dangerousness, Italy, Spain, and Sweden use the need for psychiatric treatment as the crucial criterion qualifying a person for compulsory admission. Denmark, Finland, Greece, Ireland, Portugal, and the United Kingdom use the combination of serious mental disorder and dangerousness or serious mental disorder and a need for treatment. France does not stipulate a specific legal framework for civil commitment but has established two broad procedures for civil commitment. The first, which is known as *Hospitalization d'office*, is executed by the police for persons suffering from mental health problems and considered a danger to public safety. The second, *Hospitalization à la demanded d'un tiers*, entitles family members or other close persons to apply to have someone placed involuntarily who might be unable to ask for help or care by himself or herself (Bowers, 2014, de Stefano & Ducci, 2008, Fennell & Goldstein, 2006, Jacobsen, 2012).

Germany, which has 16 federal states, independently organizes and regulates mental health care. Consequently, each federal state provides a separate legal framework for regulating involuntary placement or treatment of the mentally ill. In Germany, the basic philosophy emphasizes human rights as well as the self-determination of mentally ill patients and demands appropriate mental health care delivery in the least restrictive setting possible. This has generated a variety of regulations or statutes across the federal states in an attempt to clarify or detail procedures for treating the mentally ill against their will. Nevertheless, despite all emphasis on need or right for treatment, the threat of harm to or by a mentally ill person marks clearly the crucial condition for civil commitment (Bowers, 2014, de Stefano & Ducci, 2008).

Countries that belong to the Commonwealth of Nations have very similar civil commitment legislation. Very broadly, a person may be admitted to and detained as an involuntary patient when they appear to be mentally ill. There must also be a need for immediate treatment and that treatment can only be obtained by admission to and detention in an approved mental health service. Furthermore, due to the person's mental illness, the person is admitted and detained to protect his or her health or safety or for the protection of the public. Civil commitment can also be sought if due to mental illness the person refuses or is unable to consent to the necessary treatment. Civil commitment can also be requested if because of mental illness and the person could not receive adequate treatment in a less restrictive manner. In Australia, mental health law is constitutionally under the state powers with each state applying different laws. Consequently, in some Australian states the person must be a danger to society or themselves, while other states only require that the person be suffering from a mental illness that requires treatment. Like Australia, New Zealand law requires that the person must be a danger to themselves or others, or be unable to care for themselves.

Every province and territory in Canada has legislation which permits individuals to be kept in a psychiatric hospital against their will. Two conditions must be satisfied: the patient must be suffering from a mental disorder or mental illness, and the patient must present a danger to self or others. If these two conditions are satisfied, the law authorizes a short period of assessment within a psychiatric facility. Generally, the assessment period is less than 72 hours. The patient may kept in hospital longer if two doctors indicate the need for continued assessment. Consistent with other parts of the world, Canadian civil commitment law gives involuntary patients the right to appeal to a tribunal for a review of their case. These tribunals can order release of the patient if it concludes that the criteria for civil committal are no longer met.

In the United Kingdom legislation is based on different parts of the country, with England and Wales following one set of statutes and Northern Ireland and Scotland providing their own laws. For England and Wales, all cases of civil commitment must be justified on the basis that the individual has a serious mental disorder and that they pose a risk to harm themselves or others. Additionally, there must be access to appropriate treatment in the facility that one is being committed. In Scotland, a patient with a mental disorder, who because of that mental disorder is not capable to make decisions about the provision of medical treatment, can be treated involuntarily. Civil commitment may occur when it is a matter of urgency to detain the patient in a hospital for the purpose of determining what medical treatment may be required. Also, the patient may be detained in a hospital if there would be a significant risk *to the health*, safety or welfare of the patient, or to the safety of any other person. Under Northern Ireland law, the criteria for civil commitment includes that the person must be suffering from a mental disorder and that failure to detain the individual would create a substantial likelihood of serious physical harm to the individual or others (Bowers, 2014, Fennell & Goldstein, 2006).

As can be seen, civil commitment, whether in the United States, the European Union, or the Commonwealth of Nations all have similar or parallel definitions. In most areas of the world commitment laws focus on the concept of dangerousness to self or others. When dangerousness is upheld by a court, the right of refusal of treatment is ended. However, this broad understanding of civil commitment may be in trouble (Assembly, U.G., 2008, Callaghan & Ryan, 2014, Harpur, 2012). The United Nations Convention on the Rights of Persons with Disabilities (CRPD) is in direct contradiction with civil commitment or involuntary treatment laws. The CRPD is an international treaty designed to protect the rights and dignity of all persons with a disability. Mental health is seen as any other disabling condition (Assembly, U.G., 2008). As of October 2016, there were 160 signatories from 167 states and the European Union. These nations affirm they will promote, protect, and ensure the full enjoyment of human rights by persons with disabilities. Additionally, these nations will acknowledge that all individuals with disabilities have full equality under the law and full and equal members of society (Assembly, U.G., 2008, Callaghan & Ryan, 2014, Harpur, 2012). The United States is not obligated to fulfill the CRPD, as it did not ratify this document (Assembly, U.G., 2008, Callaghan & Ryan, 2014).

The CRPD states that there is no place for involuntary treatment based on any disability including the presence of mental illness. Effectively the United Nations has banned the notion of involuntary treatment (Assembly, U.G., 2008, Callaghan & Ryan, 2014, Harpur, 2012). If that reasoning is followed, all states who signed the CRPD need to revise their civil commitment laws. As a consequence, these new statutes would grant individuals with mental illness the same right to refuse treatment as those individuals making decisions about medical care. Additionally, dangerousness would not be the primary focus in civil commitment, but the emphasis would fall on the concept of capacity. A shift to capacity identifies the right of the individual to speak on their own behalf in the courts (Assembly, U.G., 2008, Callaghan & Ryan, 2014, Harpur, 2012).

According to the United Nations, legal capacity is what a human being can do within the structure of a legal system (Assembly, U.G., 2008, Callaghan & Ryan, 2014, Harpur, 2012). Legal capacity protects an individual's right to be recognized before the law and to make his or her own decisions. Legal capacity guarantees the exercise of one's rights, access to civil and juridical systems, and to speak on one's behalf. Under certain conditions, a person may be found to lack capacity. Those circumstances include if the individual is either (1) unable to comprehend and retain information regarding a decision or (2) unable to apply and evaluate that information (including appreciating its consequences) to make the decision (Assembly, U.G., 2008, Callaghan & Ryan, 2014, Harpur, 2012). When this occurs, the legal system can set up a substituted decision maker who becomes legally responsible on the person's behalf. As defined in the CRPD, capacity to make a decision is not based specially on the person but can include an individual's support system. With this perspective, autonomy is based on the individual's right to make their own decisions including refusal of treatment. Being a danger to self or others in not a reason to establish involuntary treatment (Assembly, U.G., 2008, Callaghan & Ryan, 2014, Harpur, 2012).

Capacity

Legal capacity refers to an assessment of the individual's psychological abilities to form rational decisions, specifically the individual's ability to understand, appreciate, and manipulate information and form rational decisions. Simply, capacity is defined as an individual's ability to make an informed decision. A licensed mental health (usually a psychiatrist) can often make a determination of capacity by focusing on an assessment of a person's mental status and its potential for interfering with specific areas of functioning. An individual who lacks capacity to make an informed decision or give consent may need to be referred for a competency hearing or need to have a guardian appointed (Callaghan & Ryan, 2014, Harpur, 2012, Grisso & Appelbaum, 1995).

The term capacity is frequently mistaken for competency. Capacity is determined by a physician (often although not exclusively by a psychiatrist) or other mental health professional, and not the courts. A patient who lacks capacity cannot exercise the right to choose or refuse treatment, and require another individual to make decisions on their behalf. The capacity to make a competent, informed decision on an issue at hand needs to be specifically considered and usually within the court system. A patient's mental status or diagnosis is not relevant to their ability to comprehend and make voluntary, informed decisions regarding the immediate problem (Callaghan & Ryan, 2014, Harpur, 2012).

Competence

Competence refers to the degree of mental soundness necessary to make decisions about a specific issue or to carry out a specific act. Competency as a legal term refers to individuals having sufficient ability and possessing the requisite natural or legal qualifications to engage in a given endeavor (Callaghan & Ryan, 2014, Harpur,

2012, Grisso & Appelbaum, 1995). Unfortunately, this broad view includes many legally recognized activities, such as the ability to enter into a contract, to stand trial, and to make medical decisions. Simply put, competency refers to the mental ability and cognitive capabilities required to execute a legally recognized act rationally (Callaghan & Ryan, 2014, Harpur, 2012, Grisso & Appelbaum, 1995). All adults are presumed to be competent unless adjudicated otherwise by a court

Incompetence, on the other hand, is related to one's functional deficits (e.g., mental illness, mental retardation, or other mental condition). These deficits must be judged sufficiently critical to undermine the potential outcomes of an individual's decision making in a specific situation (Grisso & Appelbaum, 1995). Incompetence is always decided by the court. When it is determined the individual cannot make judicious decisions on their own behalf, the court will assign surrogate (usually a guardian) to make decisions on the person's behalf (Callaghan & Ryan, 2014, Harpur, 2012, Grisso & Appelbaum, 1995).

However, the CRPD questions judgments regarding competence or capacity. This document recognizes that all people have capacity and that involuntary treatment based on medical necessity or best interest of the individual must end. Civil commitment or involuntary treatment relies on the view of substituted decision making. Substitute decision maker (SDM) is a broad term for a person appointed or identified to make health care decisions on behalf of an individual whose decision-making capability is impaired (i.e., an eating disorder). The SDM may be chosen by the person informally or formally (i.e., advanced directive). A substituted decision maker can be formally appointed by the person under the state's legal framework or it can be assigned to the person or appointed for the person by a court (Assembly,

U.G., 2008, Callaghan & Ryan, 2014, Harpur, 2012, Grisso & Appelbaum, 1995).

Involuntary treatment is generally not based on competence but capacity. It is important to remember that if the person is competent, then the substitute decision maker does not have a role. Competence is a legal matter while capacity is not. A new model that may be a better approach is called supportive decision making (Gooding, 2013). Supportive decision making works to promote self-determination, autonomy and foster independence. Supportive decision making is a process in which supporters help adult persons with mental health problems or intellectual disabilities in making decisions for their personal lives, health, financial issues, and property (Gooding, 2013). The supported persons choose independently their supporters by including members of their families, friends, and advocates they trust. This model is supported by the CRPD and is to be instituted for those who signed the CRPD (Assembly, U.G., 2008, Callaghan & Ryan, 2014, Harpur, 2012, Gooding, 2013). A key principle of supported decision making makes the supported person the most important and at the center of his/her right to choose (Gooding, 2013). Additional principles include that participation in the support network is voluntary; respect for the individual's decisions including who they want as their supporters; and that the trusted relationship between the supported person and his/her supporters is needed. The supportive decision maker organizes the startup of the network and is responsible for its sustainable development in time and avoids conflict of interests between supported persons and supporters. The model is very similar to the concept of advanced psychiatric directives, an approach that is just beginning to gain traction in the field of mental health law (Assembly, U.G., 2008, Callaghan & Ryan, 2014, Harpur, 2012, Gooding, 2013).

Civil Commitment With Individuals With Eating Disorders

Civil commitment as an approach to providing treatment is not without its critics or controversies, and a host of ethical concerns accompanies the use of civil commitment. Among the most debated ethical concerns are showing respect for the patients' autonomy (allowing patients to make their own decisions), nonmaleficence ("do no harm"), beneficence (providing care that will benefit the patient), and paternalism (interfering with a person's freedom for his or her own good). Each of these principles adds a confounding dimension to the idea of involuntary treatment. This is especially complicated when treating individuals with eating disorders that do not obviously or grossly impact the individual's reality testing (Testa & West, 2010). Along with ethical considerations are the legal aspects of civil commitment. In the United States, the prevailing standard for civil commitment is the presence of dangerousness as a result of a mental disease. The standard that most states invoke when considering civil commitment is based on the Supreme Court's criteria for holding an individual in a hospital against their will. Basically, an individual needs to have a diagnosed mental illness and be a known danger to self or harm to others (Ferris, 2008, Grace & Hardt, 2008).

Eating disorders, especially anorexia nervosa (AN), can pose serious physical and mental health risks, especially for untreated patients who fail to understand the seriousness of the disorder. The health risks for individuals who go untreated is pervasive and can adversely affect numerous organ systems with potential long-term and irreversible consequences. Untreated, these disorders can become chronic conditions interfering with an individual's ability to effectively develop normal social, psychological, academic, and occupational goals. The mortality rate for patients who develop anorexia nervosa is nearly six times the rate in the general population (Arcelus, Mitchell, Wales, & Nielsen, 2011). Additionally, AN can have one of the highest rates of death among psychiatric disorders, further putting those individuals who go untreated at risk (Harris & Barraclough, 1998). Inherent in the disorder is an inability or denial to understand the nature or seriousness of the disorder to the point that treatment refusal can threaten the total well-being of the individual. The consequence of these risks factors can lead to civil commitment. Civil commitment (compulsory treatment) must be considered and implemented when, in the judgment of the treating clinician, the individual no longer has the awareness to assist in their own care or treatment (APA, 2006).

Understanding the consequences of their actions and an ability to ascertain the seriousness of their condition, both medically and psychologically, make individuals with an eating disorder very complex when questioning their capacity. Many individuals who develop an eating disorder have what appear to be successful lives with jobs, social networks, and relationships. However, in certain circumstances their apparent inability to see the seriousness or danger of their beliefs and actions create a conflict of how to assist when the disorder overwhelms the psychological and physical condition. In that dilemma a consideration of civil commitment may occur. Although the law often is clear on the criteria what is not as well understood is whether this approach to treatment will be or benefit in both the short and long-term.

Modern Civil Commitment

At the present time, every state in the United States has a statute permitting persons to be committed because they pose a danger to themselves or others (Treatment Advocacy Center, 2013). However, after the *Donaldson* decision (Stavis, 1989), seven jurisdictions created special standards. Iowa law permits commitment when serious emotional injury could occur to family members or others who cannot avoid contact with the patient. Arizona permits commitment for persistent and acute mental disability, while Hawaii permits commitment for those obviously mentally ill. Delaware, South Carolina, and New York civil commitment statutes authorize civil commitment to inpatient care when the patient is unaware of that need. Oklahoma law focuses on the need for inpatient treatment when there has been a previous diagnosis and history of mental illness or to prevent progressive debilitation of mental illness. Twenty-three jurisdictions require commitment to be in a least restrictive setting (Stavis, 1989).

In the mid–1950s, the Supreme Court greatly enhanced personal constitutional rights especially individuals encountering any kind of incarceration by criminal sentence or civil commitment. In 1975 the Supreme Court issued a ruling regarding a state's power to civilly commit a person for psychiatric care and treatment. With *O'Connor v. Donaldson*, the requirements and limitations of due process were established (Stavis, 1989, Isaac & Brakel, 1992, Testa & West, 2010). This decision changed the constitutional principles of due process for civil commitment and seemingly merged the two previously distinct powers of civil commitments, that is, police power and the *parens patriae* power (Stavis, 1989, Testa & West, 2010). Another consequence was a greater emphasis on the concept of dangerousness when considering civil commitment with court's supporting involuntary treatment when the person is deemed dangerous to self or others. According to the Supreme Court, a state cannot constitutionally confine a non-dangerous individual who is capable of surviving safely in freedom by himself or with the help of willing and responsible family members or friends (Isaac & Brakel, 1992, Testa & West, 2010). A focus on dangerousness as the primary driver of civil commitment has created uncertainty and weakened the state's ability to act appropriately and swiftly to assist an impaired individual (Isaac & Brakel, 1992, Testa & West, 2010).

Another focus in civil commitment has been on whether an individual is able to care for oneself. This concept has become a near equivalent to dangerousness (Appelbaum & Rumpf, 1998). What this means, practically speaking, is that the courts have been redefining incapacity to care for oneself as equivalent to being a danger, or conversely expanding dangerousness to also mean being endangered (Appelbaum & Rumpf, 1998) It would certainly be easier to resurrect the *parens patriae* civil commitment statutes through the use of concepts such as gravely disabled. The use of civil commitment statutes with individuals with an eating disorder suggests that when their behavior endangers their lives, they will usually be committable under grave disability standards. This appears to comport with the practices of experts in the treatment of anorexia, and with practices in other countries as well (Appelbaum & Rumpf, 1998). Many individuals who are severely ill with an eating disorder lack competence or capacity to make treatment decisions on their own behalf, leading to involuntary treatment if necessary. Civil commitment as a method of intervention needs to be considered under circumstances that a therapeutic gain is likely from hospitalization. Civil commitment and involuntary commitment need to be considered as approach of last resort, when patients decline voluntary hospitalization and their physical safety is at risk. Civil commitment is a valid and legitimate tool to assist in the treatment of eating disorders (Appelbaum & Rumpf, 1998).

References

American Psychiatric Association. (2006). Treatment of patients with eating disorders (3rd ed.). *American Journal of Psychiatry*, 163(7 Suppl), 4–54.

Anfang, S.A., & Appelbaum, P.S. (2006). Civil commitment—the American experience. *Israel Journal of Psychiatry and Related Sciences*, 43(3), 209.

Appelbaum, P.S. (2006). History of civil commitment and related reforms in the United States: Lessons for today. *Developments in Mental Health Law*, 25, 13.

Appelbaum, P.S., & Rumpf, T. (1998). Civil commitment of the anorexic patient. *General Hospital Psychiatry*, 20(4), 225–230.

Arcelus, J., Mitchell, A.J., Wales, J., & Nielsen, S. (2011). Mortality rates in patients with anorexia nervosa and other eating disorders: A meta-analysis of 36 studies. *Archives of General Psychiatry*, 68(7), 724–731.

Assembly, U.G. (2008). Convention on the rights of persons with disabilities. *GA Res*, 61, 106.

Bloom, J.D. (2004). Thirty-five years of working with civil commitment statutes. *Journal of the American Academy of Psychiatry and the Law Online*, 32(4), 430–439.

Bowers, W.A. (2014). Civil commitment in the treatment of eating disorders and substance abuse: Empirical status and ethical considerations. In *Eating disorders, addictions and substance use disorders* (pp. 649–664). Berlin: Springer.

Callaghan, S.M., & Ryan, C. (2014). Is there a future for involuntary treatment in rights-based mental health law? *Psychiatry, Psychology and Law*, 21(5), 747–766.

de Stefano, A., & Ducci, G. (2008). Involuntary admission and compulsory treatment in Europe: An overview. *International Journal of Mental Health*, 37(3), 10–21

Fennell, P., & Goldstein, R.L. (2006). The application of civil commitment law and practices to a case of delusional disorder: A cross-national comparison of legal approaches in the United States and the United Kingdom. *Behavioral Sciences and the Law*, 24(3), 385–406.

Ferris, C.E. (2008). The search for due process in civil commitment hearings: How procedural realities have altered substantive standards. *Vanderbilt Law Review*, 61, 959.

Geller, J.L. (2006). The evolution of outpatient commitment in the USA: From conundrum to quagmire. *International Journal of Law and Psychiatry*, 29, 234–248.

Gooding, P. (2013). Supported decision-making: A rights-based disability concept and its implications for mental health law. *Psychiatry, Psychology and Law*, 20(3), 431–451.

Grace, P.J., & Hardt, E.J. (2008). When a patient refuses assistance. *American Journal of Nursing*, 108(8), 36–38.

Grisso, T., & Appelbaum, P.S. (1995). Comparison of standards for assessing patients' capacities to make treatment decisions. *American Journal of Psychiatry*, 152(7), 1033.

Harpur, P. (2012). Embracing the new disability rights paradigm: The importance of the convention on the rights of persons with disabilities. *Disability & Society*, 27(1), 1–14.

Harris, E.C., & Barraclough, B. (1998). Excess mortality of mental disorder. *British Journal of Psychiatry*, 173(1), 11–53.

Honig, J., & Stefan, S. (2005). New research continues to challenge the need for outpatient commitment. *New England Journal on Criminal and Civil Confinement*, 31, 109.

Isaac, R.J., & Brakel, S.J. (1992). Subverting good intentions: A brief history of mental health law reform. *Cornell Journal of Law and Public Policy*, 2, 89. 102–112.

Jacobsen, T.B. (2012). Involuntary treatment in Europe: Different countries, different practices. *Current Opinion in Psychiatry*, 25(4), 307–310.

Stavis, P.F. (1989). Involuntary hospitalization in the modern era: Is dangerousness ambiguous or obsolete? *Quality of Care Newsletter*, 41, 3–4.

Testa, M., & West, S.G. (2010). Civil commitment in the United States. *Psychiatry (Edgmont)*, 7, 30–40.

Treatment Advocacy Center. (2013, January). State standards for assisted treatment: Civil commitment criteria for inpatient and outpatient psychiatric treatment. Retrieved from www.treat mentadvocacycenter.org

3

Civil Commitment and Eating Disorders

Individuals with an eating disorder create challenges in the context of civil commitment and involuntary hospitalization (Kaye, 2009). For clinicians who treat these individuals, there are challenging and complicated decisions as to the best choice of care. Denial of illness and need for treatment and refusal to engage in treatment that prevents physical and psychological intervention are factors that can contribute to the deliberation for civil commitment in a small group of people with an eating disorder (Appelbaum & Rumpf, 1998). Despite the life-threatening nature of the disorder, and the best setting to restore weight is an inpatient unit, the utilization of civil commitment of individuals with eating disorders is infrequent (Brunner, Parzer, & Resch, 2005, Watson, Bowers, & Andersen, 2000). The literature on treatment of eating disorders rarely mentions its use, and the *Practice Guidelines on Eating Disorders* published by the American Psychiatric Association gives no concrete guidelines on commitment of patients with eating disorders (Brooks, 2007, Appelbaum & Rumpf, 1998, APA, 2006). Also, how mental health workers view civil commitment is different for adults and adolescents. Mental health workers who specialize in treating adults often support civil commitment regardless of the patient's decision-making capacity while those who would work with adolescents back involuntary treatment only when decision-making capacity is impaired.

Hospitalization is contemplated when an individual with an eating disorder becomes unstable with significant medical impairment such as electrolyte imbalance or cardiac problems. Psychological disruption including self-harm or suicidal ideation, social disruption or impairment on one's personal life, family distress, and occupational disruption can be factors that lead to contemplation of civil commitment (Clausen & Jones, 2014). Additional factors that lead to consideration of involuntary hospitalization are a lack of response to a reasonable trial of outpatient treatment, a need for 24-hour structured multi-disciplinary care (psychological, behavioral, and medical), and/or lack of family support or environmental toxicity (APA, 2006).

Russell (2001) points to the importance of establishing a balance between the patients' rights and their right to receive the best treatment when considering civil commitment. Of utmost importance is that family be actively involved in the care of the patient and the development of a realistic treatment plan. Following the concept of informed consent, this discussion must include the potential risks and benefits of current treatment and any information about what outcomes could occur if treatment is not intensified or discontinued. If the outcome of no treatment is a continued deterioration of health and/or a threat to one's life, then compulsory intervention is warranted. When possible, contact the family about their thoughts when civil commitment is being considered (Andersen, 2007).

The individual's ability of make competent decision regarding treatment making must be considered when considering civil commitment. Important issues include making rational decisions concerning nutritional needs, restoration of body weight and other medical treatments such as a more structured level of care (inpatient treatment) or the use of medication. The need for civil commitment then becomes important when two factors occur. One is the presence of a severe and debilitating illness together with the sustained refusal of the necessary treatment which will lead to grave physical and/or psychological impairment.

Support of civil commitment and the use of involuntary treatment indicates that the health care professional recognizes the severity of the disorder including the potential long-term impairment and how hard it can be to alter the life-threatening course of illness. Involuntary treatment can point out that collaboration between the health care provider and patient is paramount to overcome fear related to change in weight, shape, size, and appearance that inhibits successful treatment (Bowers, 2014). The literature suggests that patients and their families experience relief (albeit temporarily) when accountability for care is transferred to the professional treatment team. This shift in responsibility from the family to the professional helps guide decision making about health that is distorted by the eating disorder (Ramsay, Ward, Treasure, & Russell, 1999). In essence, it may be necessary to impose treatment (civil commitment) in order to save the life of the patient, and civil commitment can be seen as an act of compassion (Andersen, 2007).

As can be seen, an ED can be a debilitating, paralyzing, and life-threatening problem. Although some patients understand the risk of disorder and that they are ill, these patients are reluctant to accept treatment even when they are severely impaired. This reluctance can lead to confrontations among the patient, family, and clinician. When the safety of the individual clashes with their desire for maintaining the status quo or the individual is incapacitated due to the consequences of an ED, a discussion of involuntary treatment must be considered. Whether the individual is driven by their sense of autonomy, a desire to maintain self-control, or an inability to see the nature of their disorder, the clinician must make decisions intended to prevent further deterioration of the individual's health and well-being. Failure of the individual to accept the intervention leads to civil commitment using existing legal standards to compel treatment.

Instituting civil commitment suggests more of an intense or severe form of the disorder and a lack of acceptance or refusal of treatment (Ramsay et al., 1999). Individuals treated on an involuntarily basis often display differences when compared to voluntary patients. These differences include more frequent hospitalizations, a longer duration of the illness, and significantly longer time in hospital. Also, the involuntary patient has significantly more comorbid psychiatric diagnoses, more self-harm, physical or sexual abuse, and a lower age of illness onset. Civilly committed patients have higher mortality rates, lower body mass indexes (BMIs), and display greater interpersonal disruption than individuals treated voluntarily. Also, those treated on an involuntary basis took longer to reach their "target" weight (Ramsay et al., 1999, Watson et al., 2000, Ayton, Keen, & Lask, 2009, Carney, Wakefield, Tait, & Touyz, 2006). However, when compared to those voluntarily treated, patients admitted involuntarily displayed equal or greater weight restoration at discharge from hospital (Clausen & Jones, 2014).

There are concerns that the use of civil commitment will adversely influence an outpatient treatment. Some authors suggest that civil commitment creates irreparable damage to an inpatient or outpatient therapeutic relationship (Draper, 2000). Others suggest there is no loss of therapeutic relationship with health care providers (Serfaty & McCluskey, 1998). Support for this idea is buoyed by the fact that response to treatment is equal between committed and voluntary patients with no apparent loss of therapeutic relationship with their health care providers (Ramsay et al., 1999, Serfaty & McCluskey, 1998). A firm validation of the individual's safety needs and sensitive listening can enhance the therapeutic relationship during and after civil commitment. Also, patients treated against their will often say civil commitment was important after the fact (Ramsay et al., 1999, Guarda et al., 2007, Watson et al., 2000). While civil commitment may be appropriate for the very ill patient and may be essential to prevent death, it can also change a worsening long-term outcome with no effect on the therapeutic relationship (Guarda et al., 2007, Watson et al., 2000).

Patient View of Civil Commitment

Some patients deny the need for treatment initially but later agree that civil commitment was important and helpful. These individuals felt that the approach was justified and that it prevented serious medical problems and death. Some involuntarily treated patients were at such a low weight they could not make good decisions regarding their own well-being (Guarda et al., 2007, Watson et al., 2000). Patients declared civil commitment as important early in treatment to prevent the disorder from becoming more chronic in nature. Patients suggest that the important aspect of civil commitment is not the involuntary treatment but how the individual is treated during and after being civilly committed (Tan, Hope, Stewart, & Fitzpatrick, 2003, Elzakkers, Danner, Hoek, Schmidt, & Elburg, 2014). Any sense of coercion was related to the relationship between the patient and the mental health professions (Tan et al., 2003, Elzakkers et al., 2014). Although some patients saw civil commitment as a factor to continue engagement in treatment, other patients felt involuntary treatment should be reserved only for situations that were considered life-threatening (Tan et al., 2003, Elzakkers et al., 2014).

The need for lifesaving interventions creates numerous dilemmas for professionals who treat these disorders. The literature does not offer good data on outcome of civil commitment but there is some guidance when looking at AN. The limited empirical data, although contradictory in nature, suggest that involuntary treatment is beneficial (Andersen, 2007). It appears that a relatively small proportion of the ED population is severely ill enough to be detained for treatment. Patients admitted involuntarily range from 1.5% to 11.6% in the United Kingdom while data from other countries indicate a range from 8% (in Ireland) to 28% (in Australia). Watson et al. (2000) indicated that 16.6% ($N = 66$ of 397) of patients admitted to a hospital for specialized treatment warranted civil commitment. There is other data suggesting that specialized treatment programs civilly commit between 20% and 35% of their patients (Elzakkers et al., 2014).

Patients with anorexia nervosa treated on an inpatient basis reported a stronger sense of coercion (Tan et al., 2003). Treatment of individuals via civil commitment reported more negative events such as nasogastric feedings, refeeding syndrome, and more coercive environment such as a locked hospital unit. One 5-year follow-up of involuntary patients suggested that for severe cases it appeared that treatment was of marginal benefit (Ben-Tovim et al., 2001).

Ramsay et al. (1999) confirmed that short-term treatment of involuntary and voluntary patients are comparably effective, but the long-term outcome is more problematic for involuntary patients, with mortality rates being higher at 5.5-year follow-up (Ramsay et al., 1999). When compared to voluntary treated patients, involuntary patients had a higher mortality rate (3% vs. 13%) (Tan et al., 2003). Although weight restoration was equivalent between voluntary and involuntary patients, there was a slower rate of restoration for involuntary patients (Watson, et al., 2000). A high mortality rate and overall interference of functioning for individuals with an eating disorder creates conflict for the health care provider on how or when to use civil commitment as a method to facilitate patient health. Conflicting long-term outcome with involuntary treatment suggests that involuntarily treated patients had better general functioning and normalization of weight than voluntarily treated patients (Elzakkers et al., 2014).

Persuasion vs. Coercion

Power is a fact of daily life, just as various forms of coercion are a (controversial) companion in the treatment of severe anorexia nervosa (Andersen, 2007). Forms of strong persuasion, browbeating, or even outright moral blackmail are deployed in many social contexts (including in the treatment of eating disorders; Guarda et al., 2007). Coercion can be applied in many settings or across a continuum of care. Some power differentials are magnified (such as inpatient care), while in community-based care (outpatient care) or professional relationships the power differentials are much more nuanced (Carney et al., 2007). It might be safe to say that involuntary treatment or civil commitment is the ultimate in coercion.

In most areas of medicine, individuals have the right to make their own decisions even if those decisions may be seen as irrational, idiosyncratic, or unreasonable. The exception in medicine occurs with those individuals identified with psychiatric disorders. The nature of eating disorders symptoms impedes the individual from completely understanding how the disorder interferes with decision making. This interference often leads to conflict among family, significant others, professionals, and patients focusing on how to intervene with a potential life-threatening problem. It is in the midst of this conflict that individuals with an eating disorder often report high levels of "perceived coercion" to engage in treatment. The coercion can occur with or without formal or legal intervention. However, threat of legal intervention is identified as one form of coercion that contributes to engagement in treatment or admission to a hospital (Andersen, 2007, Bowers, 2014, Tan et al., 2003).

Research shows that only 9%–28% of patients are actually hospitalized via legal methods. This may seem like a low number when considering civil commitment as a pathway to inpatient care, especially for individuals with anorexia nervosa. However, patients with anorexia nervosa treated on an inpatient basis report a stronger sense of coercion (Tan et al., 2003). Civil commitment is also seen as highly stigmatizing, reinforcing a perceived loss of freedom of decision making, leading to a sense of being dismissed, belittled, or treated punitively by health care professionals. From a patient perspective, civil commitment is seen as the worst option to engage in treatment compared to other forms of leverage employed by health care professionals or families (Tan et al., 2003).

In most countries, mental health professionals are legally empowered to act paternalistically to override treatment refusal by patients with mental disorders using either mental health law or child welfare statutes. Treatment without patient consent, even if legally permitted by mental health legislation, may be ethically difficult to justify if patients are unimpaired in their ability to make valid treatment decisions (Draper, 2000, Dresser, 1984a, 1984b). Some patients strongly suggest that enforced treatment directly affects their ability to make balanced decisions with respect to immediate or long-term care. Compulsory treatment was viewed as inflicting suffering, prison, and punishment. Mothers and daughters who perceived civil commitment as life-sustaining also saw it as a negative experience. Civil commitment has been characterized as being equivalent to imprisonment and punishment. This negative perception raises the issue of whether such treatment, however effective, is morally permissible and whether it is infringing the right of a person to make medical decisions (Tan et al., 2003). It can be hard to take control over an individual's decision making without help or support from significant others. Patients have noted that returning control and choice was crucial in empowering a decision to accept treatment.

Civil commitment and overriding autonomy is justified when it saves a life (Andersen, 2007, Bowers, 2014). However, patients find that the struggle for control has a powerful impact on their ability to accept treatment which has implications for the issue of civil commitment. Other implications include: Is civil commitment more appropriate for adults who do not have the support of their parents? Does this type of intervention need to be implemented much earlier in treatment rather than at the stage to save a life? Does civil commitment keep the patient focused, or can it be a motivator to help the patient remain focused on the seriousness of the disorder? Currently these questions have not been addressed or tested empirically. Indirectly, we know that some involuntarily committed patients who initially objected to their commitment had positive views of their hospitalization. At discharge, these individuals stated they would want to be hospitalized in the future if they became dangerously ill again (Guarda et al., 2007, Watson et al., 2000). Also, at the end of inpatient care many involuntary patients report an understanding of and gave support to the need for treatment (Guarda et al., 2007, Watson et al., 2000). Perhaps we need to look at civil commitment as a part of our overall treatment plan rather than just to save lives. No one should die when a disorder is treatable.

Civil commitment is open to criticism as it strips the person of their right to choose and exercise autonomy even if foolish decisions are being made. However, in hindsight, some patients were thankful and saw civil commitment as justified. This was especially true if it was necessary to maintain life (Guarda et al., 2007, Watson et al., 2000). This is hard when implementing involuntary care. However, patients identified successful treatment was best when patients were included in all treatment decision making. Context and relationships within which treatment decisions are made are critical to the patient's view of choice or compulsion for treatment. Freedom of choice is often less important than the relationships and attitudes of family and health care workers. Civil commitment is seen as helpful and caring by some individuals. Leverage or forced treatment can be deemed acceptable if there is a shared and respected relationship between the care provider and the patient (Tan et al., 2003, Tan, Hope, Stewart, & Fitzpatrick, 2006, Tan & Richards, 2015).

Civil commitment is acceptable in order to save a life. Is then involuntary or coercive treatment justified in treating ED? When poor insight and the probable ego-syntonic nature of ED lead to treatment refusal and the potential for life-threatening outcomes, then the answer is yes! However, treatment to preserve health often violates the patients' desire for autonomy leading to an inherently paternalistic approach to care. The patients' response to involuntary weight restoration or forced treatment (paternalistic care) can lead to a strong sense of coercion on the part of the patient. In fact, even in voluntary admissions to an inpatient unit, patients perceive coercive pressure from clinicians, family, friends, employers, or educators. Research suggests individuals with more frequent involuntary hospitalizations indicated that they were more resistant to treatment with 35% of patients admitted to an ED specialty unit denying the need for admission (Guarda et al., 2007, Watson et al., 2000). Similarly these patients reported a significantly higher level of perceived coercion and pressure for admission by others than did patients who spontaneously requested admission. Researchers (Bindman et al., 2005, Rain et al., 2003, Swartz et al., 1999) have also found that patients legally committed for involuntary treatment tend to hold more negative views of their hospitalization than patients admitted for voluntary treatment and report at discharge that little or no benefit has occurred. Ramsay et al. (1999) reported that involuntary commitment of patients with AN led to satisfactory short-term treatment results but increased long-term morbidity. The mortality at follow-up for the detained patients was 12.7%, compared to 2.6% for the voluntary patients. In contrast, other researchers (Guarda et al., 2007, Watson et al., 2000) have found that most involuntarily committed patients who initially objected to their commitment had positive views of their hospitalization and treatment at discharge and would want to be hospitalized in the future if they became dangerously ill again. Also, at the end of inpatient care many involuntary patients reported an understanding of and gave support to the need for treatment. These data reinforce involuntary treatment for some seriously ill patients (Watson et al., 2000). Additionally, the shift in initial resistance to treatment suggests that the patient's unrealistic beliefs are directly related to the disorder (Guarda et al., 2007, Watson et al., 2000). Nevertheless, for selected cases of individuals with ED that is life-threatening and associated with denial of illness, a court-imposed use of involuntary treatment may be appropriate (Watson et al., 2000).

Compulsory treatment can be viewed as being in the best interest of the patient, family, and care provider. It is a serious decision that often creates a great deal of angst among the treatment providers and family. For the patient, civil commitment offers the opportunity to continue in treatment and work toward both physical and psychological wellness. The benefits for the health care professional include a means to address life-threatening medical and psychological problems when the patient does not agree with a professional's assessment. Equally important, civil commitment can provide the family or significant other with reduced emotional distress and reduce the stress of feeling scared or "trapped" regarding the health of their loved one. Compulsory treatment may be of crucial importance preventing death of patients with chronic anorexia nervosa and psychiatric comorbidities (Andersen, 2007, Yager, Carney, & Touyz, 2016). Delayed treatment in children and adolescents may lead to medical complications such as stunted growth, delayed menses, or cessation of menstrual periods. Additionally, delayed treatment may affect adolescent relationships with parents and peers, distorted self-perception, lowered self-esteem, and difficulty forming close relationships (APA 2006, Strober, Freeman, & Morrell, 1997).

On the other end of the continuum, civil commitment is viewed as violating the individual's right to decide (autonomy). It has been suggested that civil commitment does not treat the disorder, as successful treatment requires patient cooperation. Some authors strongly suggest that civil commitment creates lasting damage to the therapeutic relationship, reducing the desire to remain in treatment. One criticism of civil commitment is that when improvement in the disorder does not occur past medical stabilization, there is no long-term positive outcome. Conflicting opinions exist regarding any involuntary treatment of a psychiatric disorder, especially AN. A review of the involuntary commitment literature (Hiday, 1996, Swartz et al., 1999) found that two hypotheses guide outcome studies of involuntary legal commitment. One hypothesis predicts that involuntary patients will be angry and negative about their hospitalization and treatment. Thus, they will be less likely to cooperate in the hospital and in the community, thus resulting in rehospitalization. The other hypothesis predicts that the initial anger and negativism of involuntary patients will subside and that they will become positive toward their hospitalization and treatment after they receive help.

There is a need to better understand the ethics, role, and outcome of legal and non-legal forms of leveraged treatment (Schreyer et al., 2016). Civil commitment can be seen as compassionate care. If the medical and psychiatric condition of the patient meets the legal criteria for involuntary treatment, there is no reason individuals with an eating disorder should be discounted from lifesaving treatment. Short-term beneficence and paternalism trumps autonomy in selected situations, as long as autonomy is restored with treatment (Andersen, 2007, Bowers, 2014, Caplan, 2006). The need for involuntary treatment is often perceived as coercive. However, this approach is validated by the serious nature of the eating disorder. Paternalism or the perception of coercion does not endure for long. Improvement in the patient can strengthen therapeutic alliance with the treatment team leading to a return of autonomy. When long-term aspects of mandated treatment are examined, the less favorable outcome for the involuntarily treated patient was not a direct consequence of the acute involuntary treatment itself (Andersen, 2007, Bowers, 2014, Caplan, 2006).

Outpatient Civil Commitment

Outpatient civil commitment is a relatively modern trend. It is designed to allow people suffering from mental disorders to remain in their communities. It mandates the treatment of individuals who could potentially become dangerous to themselves or others without forcing them to be hospitalized. When a psychiatrically ill individual has a pattern of deteriorating and becoming dangerous away from treatment, it is in the patient's and public interest to intervene early. States with early intervention statutes rely on the concept of grave disability which has merit with an individual with an eating disorder (Treatment Advocacy Center, 2013). Outpatient commitment statutes that focus on grave disability can move away from the dangerousness concept that dominates civil commitment law.

The chronic starvation or binge/purge behavior of an individual with an eating disorder may not be considered suicidal behavior, yet these actions if they go unchecked can lead to threat to life. State civil commitment laws are designed to ensure that persons with mental illness get the needed treatment when they become a danger to self or others (West & Friedman, 2010). In the case of an individual with an eating disorder, state statutes could allow for commitment of patients whose behavior renders them gravely disabled, which could lead to life-threatening consequences if unchecked. The actions or inactions of the patient can be deemed so disabling as to create an imminent risk of harm. Unfortunately, there is no consensus even among eating disorder specialists as to what clinical signs indicate imminent risk to self (Appelbaum & Rumpf, 1998).

Another use of outpatient commitment is when inpatient care has reached its goals. The addition of outpatient care becomes paramount to maintain early treatment goals and continue healing. In most states outpatient commitment statutes exist to continue monitoring the health of the individual (West & Friedman, 2010, Anfang & Appelbaum, 2006). In general, outpatient civil commitment depends on several criteria. First, the individual considered for outpatient commitment must be diagnosed with a mental disorder. Second, the individual needs to clearly be in need of continued treatment and have a history of inadequate awareness regarding their need for continuation of treatment. A pattern of nonadherence to treatment indicates that the patient would not reliably access psychiatric care on a voluntary basis. Third, there must be evidence indicating that the individual is likely to decompensate into a state that would prove dangerous to him or herself or others if treatment nonadherence were to occur (Anfang, & Appelbaum 2006). If the criteria are met, the individual can be mandated to outpatient psychiatric treatment (West & Friedman, 2010, Anfang & Appelbaum, 2006).

The benefit of outpatient commitment is that it increases the likelihood of continued supervising of any exacerbation of the disorder. Additionally, it requires adherence to treatment and early intervention if needed. Individuals under outpatient civil commitment are easier to rehospitalize when deterioration of their illness occurs. Families also often find it easier to access needed care for mentally ill relatives who are subject to outpatient commitment (Copeland & Heilemann 2008). Additionally, outpatient commitment has been shown to be effective in improving patients' psychiatric outcomes, decreasing rates of hospitalization and lengths of inpatient psychiatric stays, and increasing participation in community psychiatric treatment (Segal & Burgess, 2009).

Where outpatient commitment is implemented, the following standards are advised to maintain the individual's autonomy. Outpatient commitment should not last longer than the law requires and be based on current evidence of dangerousness to self or others or grave disability. The least restrictive level of care must be honored during involuntary treatment and no coercion should be implemented to lengthen involuntary status. Involuntary treatment should be based on a significant history of nonresponsiveness to community care, and failure to comply with treatment need not be the sole standard for revocation of outpatient status or recommitment. Return to a more intense level of care and involuntary care must be based on dangerousness to self or others (Testa & West, 2010).

References

American Psychiatric Association. (2006). Treatment of patients with eating disorders (3rd ed.). *American Journal of Psychiatry*, 163(7 Suppl), 4–54.

Anfang, S.A., & Appelbaum, P.S. (2006). Civil commitment—the American experience. *Israel Journal of Psychiatry and Related Sciences*, 43(3), 209.

Appelbaum, P.S., & Rumpf, T. (1998). Civil commitment of the anorexic patient. *General Hospital Psychiatry*, 20(4), 225–230.

Ayton, A., Keen, C., & Lask, B. (2009). Pros and cons of using the Mental Health Act for severe eating disorders in adolescents. *European Eating Disorders Review*, 17(1), 14–23.

Ben-Tovim, D.I., Walker, K., Gilchrist, P., Freeman, R., Kalucy, R., & Esterman, A. (2001). Outcome in patients with eating disorders: A 5-year study. *Lancet*, 357, 1254–1257.

Bindman, J., Reid, Y., Szmukler, G., Tiller, J., Thornicroft, G., & Leese, M. (2005). Perceived coercion at admission to psychiatric hospital and engagement with follow-up. *Social Psychiatry and Psychiatric Epidemiology*, 40(2), 160–166.

Bowers, W.A. (2014). Civil commitment in the treatment of eating disorders and substance abuse: Empirical status and ethical considerations. In *Eating disorders, addictions and substance use disorders* (pp. 649–664). Berlin: Springer.

Brooks, R.A. (2007). Psychiatrists' opinions about involuntary civil commitment: Results of a national survey. *Journal of the American Academy of Psychiatry and the Law Online*, 35(2), 219–228.

Brunner, R., Parzer, P., & Resch, F. (2005). Involuntary hospitalization of patients with anorexia nervosa: Clinical issues and empirical findings. *Fortschritte der Neurologie-Psychiatrie*, 73(1), 9–15.

Caplan, A.L. (2006). Ethical issues surrounding forced, mandated, or coerced treatment. *Journal of Substance Abuse Treatment*, 31(2), 117–120.

Carney, T., Tait, D., & Touyz, S. (2007). Coercion is coercion? Reflections on trends in the use of compulsion in treating anorexia nervosa. *Australasian Psychiatry*, 15(5), 390–395.

Carney, T., Wakefield, A., Tait, D., & Touyz, S. (2006). Reflections on coercion in the treatment of severe anorexia nervosa. *Israel Journal of Psychiatry and Related Sciences*, 43(3), 159–165.

Clausen, L., & Jones, A. (2014). A systematic review of the frequency, duration, type and effect of involuntary treatment for people with anorexia nervosa, and an analysis of patient characteristics. *Journal of Eating Disorders*, 2(1), 29.

Copeland, D.A., & Heilemann, M.V. (2008). Getting to "the point": The experience of mothers getting assistance for their violent, mentally ill, adult children. *Nursing Research*, 57(3), 136.

Draper, H. (2000). Anorexia nervosa and respecting a refusal of life-prolonging therapy: A limited justification. *Bioethics*, 14(2), 120–133.

Dresser, R. (1984a). Feeding the hunger artists: Legal issues in treating anorexia nervosa. *Wisconsin Law Review*, 297.

Dresser, R. (1984b). Legal and policy considerations in treatment of anorexia nervosa patients. *International Journal of Eating Disorders*, 3(4), 43–51.

Elzakkers, I.F., Danner, U.N., Hoek, H.W., Schmidt, U., & Elburg, A.A. (2014). Compulsory treatment in anorexia nervosa: A review. *International Journal of Eating Disorders*, 47(8), 845–852.

Guarda, A., Pinto, A., Coughlin, J., Hussain, S., Haug, N., & Heinberg, L. (2007). Perceived coercion and change in perceived need for admission in patients hospitalized for eating disorders. *American Journal of Psychiatry*, 164, 108–114.

Hiday, V.A. (1996). Involuntary commitment as a psychiatric technology. *International Journal of Technology Assessment in Health Care*, 12, 585–603.

Kaye, W. (2009). Eating disorders: Hope despite mortal risk. *American Journal of Psychiatry* (166), 1309–1311.

Rain, S.D., Williams, V.F., Robbins, P.C., Monahan, J., Steadman, H.J., & Vesselinov, R. (2003). Perceived coercion at hospital admission and adherence to mental health treatment after discharge. *Psychiatric Services*, 54, 103–105.

Ramsay, R., Ward, A., Treasure, J., & Russell, G.F. (1999). Compulsory treatment in anorexia nervosa: Short-term benefits and long-term mortality. *British Journal of Psychiatry*, 175(2), 147–153.

Russell, G.F. (2001). Involuntary treatment in anorexia nervosa. *Psychiatric Clinics of North America*, 24(2), 337–349.

Schreyer, C.C., Coughlin, J.W., Makhzoumi, S.H., Redgrave, G.W., Hansen, J.L., & Guarda, A.S. (2016). Perceived coercion in inpatients with anorexia nervosa: Associations with illness severity and hospital course. *International Journal of Eating Disorders*, 49(4), 407–412.

Segal, S.P., & Burgess, P.M. (2009). The utility of extended outpatient civil commitment. *International Journal of Law and Psychiatry*, 29(6), 525–534.

Serfaty, M., & McCluskey, S. (1998). Compulsory treatment of anorexia nervosa and the moribund patient. *European Eating Disorders Review*, 6(1), 27–37.

Strober, M., Freeman, R., & Morrell, W. (1997). The long-term course of severe anorexia nervosa in adolescents: Survival analysis of recovery, relapse, and outcome predictors over 10–15 years in a prospective study. *International Journal of Eating Disorders*, 22(4), 339–360.

Swartz, M.S., Swanson, J.W., Wagner, H.R., Burns, B.J., Hiday, V.A., & Borum, R. (1999). Can involuntary outpatient commitment reduce hospital recidivism? Findings from a randomized trial with severely mentally ill individuals. *American Journal of Psychiatry*, 156, 1968–1975.

Tan, J.O., Hope, T., Stewart, A., & Fitzpatrick, R. (2003). Control and compulsory treatment in anorexia nervosa: The views of patients and parents. *International Journal of Law and Psychiatry*, 26(6), 627–645.

Tan, J.O., Hope, T., Stewart, A., & Fitzpatrick, R. (2006). Competence to make treatment decisions in anorexia nervosa: Thinking processes and values. *Philosophy, Psychiatry, & Psychology: PPP*, 13(4), 267.

Tan, J., & Richards, L. (2015). Legal and ethical issues in the treatment of really sick patients with anorexia nervosa. In P.H. Robinson & D. Nicholls (Eds.), *Critical care for anorexia nervosa* (pp. 113–150). Switzerland: Springer.

Testa, M., & West, S.G. (2010). Civil commitment in the United States. *Psychiatry (Edgmont)*, 7, 30–40.

Treatment Advocacy Center. (2013, January). State standards for assisted treatment: Civil commitment criteria for inpatient and outpatient psychiatric treatment. Retrieved from www.treatmentadvocacycenter.org

Watson, T.L., Bowers, W.A., & Andersen, A.E. (2000). Involuntary treatment of eating disorders. *American Journal of Psychiatry*, 157, 1806–1810.

West, S.G., & Friedman, S.H. (2010). Entry on civil commitment. In *Wiley encyclopedia of forensic science—Behavioral sciences*. Hoboken, NJ: John Wiley & Sons.

Yager, J., Carney, T., & Touyz, S. (2016). Is involuntary (compulsory) treatment ever justified in patients with SE-AN: An international perspective. In S. Touyz, D. LeGrange, H. Lacey, & P. Hay (Eds.), *Managing severe and enduring anorexia nervosa: A clinician's guide* (pp. 185–201). Abingdon: Routledge.

4

Ethical Considerations

A problematic characteristic of eating disorders (ED) is the reluctance of patients to accept treatment even when they are at significant physical and psychological risk. Although these patients typically deny intent to harm themselves, their actions can result in life-threatening medical complications. Severely ill patients may lack the capacity to make competent treatment decisions, and situations may arise when lifesaving procedures are justified. There is uncertainty however around when and for whom involuntary treatment may be justified, and ethical questions can arise during consideration of compulsory treatment.

On the other end of the continuum, civil commitment is viewed as violating the individual's rights to decide (autonomy). It has been suggested that civil commitment does not treat the disorder, as successful treatment requires patient cooperation. Some authors strongly suggest that civil commitment creates lasting damage to the therapeutic relationship, reducing the desire to remain in treatment. One criticism of civil commitment is that when improvement in the disorder does not occur past medical stabilization, there is no long-term positive outcome. Conflicting opinions exist regarding any involuntary treatment of a psychiatric disorder, especially AN.

A review of the involuntary commitment literature (Hiday, 1996, Swartz et al., 1999) found that two hypotheses guide outcome studies of involuntary legal commitment. One hypothesis predicts that involuntary patients will be angry and negative about their hospitalization and treatment. They will be less likely to cooperate in the hospital and in the community, thus resulting in rehospitalization. The other hypothesis predicts that the initial anger and negativism of involuntary patients will subside and that they will become positive toward their hospitalization and treatment after they receive help.

Ethical Considerations

In most cases involving eating disorders (primarily anorexia nervosa), by the time involuntary hospitalization and treatment are under consideration, the patient will have been deemed incompetent and lacking decisional capacity. The consequence of those behaviors directs the health care provider or family toward coercion. The perception of coercion in civil commitment is complex and not necessarily related to the degree of restriction of freedom. In thinking about and invoking compulsory treatment, we want to do what is right and good or at least what will be best for the greatest number. In considering civil commitment, there needs to be a balanced, ethically principled approach that respects the dignity or autonomy of the affected person while working to prevent deterioration of the person's health. Respect for personal dignity does not rely on autonomy (allowing patients to make their own decisions) alone, but is also supported by the principles of beneficence (providing care that will benefit the patient), nonmaleficence (do no harm), and paternalism (interfering with a person's freedom for his or her own good). We recognize each of these principles as intrinsically ethical or moral. However, at some point, even the most profoundly caring provider may find themselves inclined to violate an individual's autonomy when the extent of their illness makes it impossible to maintain health. Beneficence and paternalism can be seen as overruling autonomy (Kenney, 2012, Tansey, 2011). As noted earlier, people with eating disorders, especially anorexia nervosa, appear to agree with the necessity of compulsory treatment in order to save life (Tan & Richards 2015, Tan, Hope, Stewart, & Fitzpatrick, 2003).

The decision to treat involuntarily should be subjected to the most rigorous standards. Primary questions that should be considered are (1) Is this an end of life situation? (2) How would the patient benefit from treatment? Will others benefit (i.e., family, providers, the community)? (3) How realistic are our treatment goals? (4) What criteria will constitute success or failure? (5) What time frame may be agreed upon for imposing the treatment? (6) What financial concerns are relevant for the patient or family? (7) What is our standard of care? (8) What does the medical literature suggest about the efficacy of involuntary treatment? Each question must be considered by all involved parties (Kenney, 2012).

What ethical principles do we rely upon in this decision? What makes it morally permissible, or morally repugnant? Is there a consensus for this decision? It may be morally permissible to force a person with a life-threatening mental disorder into treatment, but why? One idea that has been advanced is that the individual is no longer able to make competent decisions. Although the individual may suggest they are making a choice, poor decision making or incompetence will be influenced by impaired self-awareness or an inability to control the behaviors that are characteristic of the disorder or illness. Severe mental illness can lead to an unrealistic appraisal of the implications and consequences of the individual's actions. Respect for persons, coupled with concerns animated by beneficence, nonmaleficence, and paternalism, provide grounds for the appointment of a surrogate decision maker who can request involuntary treatment. If they decide to compel another person into treatment, this course of action must proceed with personal humility, cultural humility, professional humility, and in awe of the dignity of the human person (Kenney, 2012, Tansey, 2011).

Of primary concern in civil commitment is the principle of autonomy (Silber, 2011). Related to the individual's control over his or her body, this principle has long been a central concept in medicine. Within the substance abuse literature, there is a view that mandatory treatment involves protecting third parties from extreme health risks or those incapable of autonomy. However, when autonomy is compromised but there is a debilitating illness, there is a need to override autonomy with justified paternalism (Silber, 2011). Caplan (2006) has put forth the argument that respect for self-determination sometimes requires mandatory treatment as a way to create or enable autonomy. The premise is that people who are severely ill do not have the full capacity to be self-determined or autonomous because they are caught up in their illness. If this is indeed true, then it may be possible to justify compulsory treatment in order to return autonomy to the affected individual. Caplan (2006) also advances the idea that illness itself can be a form of coercion, as the person is driven by desires that go on to influence actions and behaviors. Physiological and psychological changes as well as fear of loss of control or weight gain are powerful motivators to continue illness behavior. If treatment can facilitate change, it will increase the individual's autonomy and their ability to maintain health. Maintaining health and the ability to make good choices about their actions in the long run would be the moral thing to do (Caplan, 2006).

A similar idea has been suggested when treating anorexia nervosa (Craigie, Hope, Tan, Stewart, & McMillan, 2013). These authors propose that the eating disorder subtly compromises autonomy, inhibiting a clear understanding of actions and decision about shape and weight that affect overall health. Looking at the experiences of individuals with AN, it was found that treatment refusal was based on emotional experiences and false beliefs that contributed to an inability to make knowledgeable decisions. As a result, competence and autonomy were significantly compromised. The ED inhibits an individual's awareness of the outcome of their actions, which in turn leads to treatment refusal. The refusal of treatment may seem autonomous but in reality is influenced by the disorder. Compulsory treatment is seen as a method to reduce ambivalence about treatment, assist in changing false beliefs about weight, shape, and health while restoring the person's autonomy to make appropriate health care decisions.

General Ethical Principles

The cornerstone of current ethics thinking in medicine is based on the principles of autonomy (freedom from external control or influence; respecting their views about a particular treatments), beneficence (balancing the benefits of treatment against the risks and costs involved), nonmaleficence (the harm should not be disproportionate to the benefit of the treatment), and justice (the moral obligation to act on the basis of fair adjudication between competing claims). Paramount to ethical consideration is the respect for the autonomy of the individual. Comprehending the ethical underpinnings (especially autonomy) is mandatory to the understanding of how they are understood in the treatment of eating disorders. When involuntary commitment is contemplated these individual values must be considered prior any decision to violate them (Tansey, 2011). Respecting the principles of beneficence and nonmaleficence may in certain circumstances mean failing to respect a person's autonomy. For example, it may be necessary to provide treatment that is not desired in order to prevent the development of a future, more serious health problem. The treatment might be unpleasant, uncomfortable, or even painful, but this might involve less harm to the patient than would occur were they not to have it (Kenney, 2012, Tansey, 2011).

When the focus is on the treatment of eating disorders, the ethical principle that is most directly related to civil commitment is the violation of one's autonomy. Autonomy conveys the idea that the individual can make their own decisions without the constraint of others. Additionally, autonomous decisions convey the idea that these choices are made from distinct and coherent thought in agreement with what the individual wants from life. Overruling an individual's right to make their own treatment decisions implies that they have lost the capacity to make judgments about their health. In the case of eating disorders, especially anorexia nervosa, good clinical care can make overriding autonomy a critical issue (Tan & Richards, 2015, Tan et al., 2003).

Andersen (2007) states that severely ill eating disorder patients often appear more competent than they actually are. They can identify how poor their physical state has become and agree that without intervention or change, they may well die. Eating disorder patients (especially those with anorexia nervosa) often appear to agree to treatment. However, this gives way to multiple reasons to delay treatment that are seemingly compelled by unsound reasoning. When deciding when a patient with an eating disorder is too ill to make an informed decision about the need for treatment, clinicians must assert the patient is too sick to be autonomous. Carefully delineated respect for both autonomy and beneficence, combined with experienced assessment of mental and behavioral functioning in AN, will determine when beneficence trumps autonomy (Andersen, 2007).

Andersen (2007) suggests that ethical principles come into conflict when considering civil commitment. It is vital the clinician understand how starvation influences the psychological and behavioral expressions that leads to the eating disorders rigid and overvalued beliefs. Also, starvation can be a maintaining factor in anorexia nervosa. The overvalued beliefs of individuals who develop an eating disorder can be seen by them and others as a positive characteristic that helps order their lives. This leads to the conviction that these individuals can make decisions in their best interest (autonomy). However, the overvalued beliefs regarding need for control and fear of weight change undermine the individual's capacity to modify actions that promote psychological impairment, physical deterioration, or death. In fact, these individuals have little voluntary control to make autonomous decisions. Any deviation from the overvalued beliefs about the disorder leads to a sense of personal failure for the individual, which leads to a more rigid stance about their beliefs, creating a vicious cycle of restriction, strategies for weight loss, and overcontrol. The very nature of this cycle lends itself to questioning how autonomous the patient really is (Andersen, 2007).

The issue of how compromised is autonomy for individuals with an eating disorder can be controversial. Though it may be apparent that decisions regarding nutrition and weight are compromised, it can seem like other areas in their lives are under the function of competent reasoning. Craigie et al. (2013) challenge this perspective and feel that individuals with eating disorders, especially anorexia nervosa, are severely compromised, and that this compromise inhibits autonomy. They posit four areas in which autonomy is compromised especially when related to eating and weight: agency, affective components, inner conflicts that influence the stability of preferences and beliefs, and intense concerns about identity and authenticity.

Craigie et al. (2013) strongly suggest that the development of an eating disorder, especially anorexia nervosa, is not a life choice that has been selected after careful consideration of the pros and cons relative to one's life goals. They imply the lives of individuals with an eating disorder have become a burden and they are no longer able, via autonomous reasoning, to obtain specific results such as eating or weight gain. The disorder has stopped the individual from exercising autonomy (agency) to get what they want from life. How do these individuals make the necessary changes (gain weight, stop purging) to reverse the problem and assert their autonomy? Helping the individual regain autonomy means for them to face their fears in order to pursue their life goals.

The fear of weight gain or being out of control has become so strong that rational decision making has become subservient to their anxiety. Fear of weight gain or eating adequate nutrition robs them of autonomous actions related to health and quality of life. When fear is so strong that it deprives the individual of autonomy, it is prudent for clinicians to override an individual's illusion of autonomy. From a treatment standpoint, autonomy is about motivating the individual to overcome her anxiety and have a better life. Ethically, the fear of change (impaired autonomy) does not necessarily suggest incompetence but rather infers reduced autonomy, which may interfere with life goals and must be addressed in treatment (Craigie et al., 2013).

Many beliefs that accompany an eating disorder do not reflect rational or objective thought. However, those beliefs influence how the individual behaves and disrupts autonomous decision making. The beliefs are embedded in strong emotional experiences which reduce the individual's ability to evaluate the consequences of their thoughts and behaviors. The drive of the individual is to reduce or eliminate their uncomfortable experience rather than being aware of how it influences actions and interferes with autonomous thinking. Autonomous actions are overwhelmed by a desire to "not feel," and rational thought and actions are abandoned. Belief is governed by emotion, not rational or autonomous thinking (Tan et al., 2003).

Emotional distress creates and maintains a vicious cycle. In an effort to not feel or reduce distress the individual maintains beliefs and engages in actions that perpetuate the disorder. Overvalued beliefs like fear of weight gain and being out of control create default actions like restricting nutritional intake or extreme food rules. The default actions create an illusion of controlling distress but never help the individual cope effectively. While the person with an eating disorder can acknowledge their conflict, the intense emotional distress overrides autonomous decision making. These individuals appear to understand the problems and consequences of an eating disorder (medical complications, disrupted interpersonal relationships, impaired life goals) but emotional distress works to maintain their beliefs and keeps engagement their behavior. Conflict between health and control, overvalued ideation about weight, shape, size and appearance creates an intense emotional state that implies that the individual is not thinking in an autonomous manner and that the individual is no longer competent to make decisions that reflect their best interest.

Bratton (2010) takes the stance that eating disorders (primarily anorexia nervosa) represent a failure of autonomy. Whether there is capacity or not, an eating disorder disrupts autonomy and interferes with self-actualization. To return the individual to autonomy there must be an improvement in one's medical condition along with a return to living a valued life. The eating disorder inhibits one's ability to make autonomous decisions about health and well-being even though other parts of a person's life seem normal. The question of capacity or competence (autonomous thinking) for an individual with an eating disorder would be based on their ability to make rational decisions (Matusek & Wright, 2010). Another way to look at this is by asking the question, would the affected individual with an eating disorder make the same decisions about what they want their life to be if they did not have this illness? Looking at the literature, the answer seems to be no (Tan et al., 2003).

Although autonomy gets the lion's share of attention when discussing ethical considerations and eating disorders, there are other aspects of ethical care that are also important. The principles of beneficence (providing care that will benefit the patient), nonmaleficence (do no harm), and justice (striving for fairness) must maintain a focus when considering civil commitment. Similarly, the duty to protect (the responsibility to protect an individuals' or other third party's welfare when they are at risk of harm) and paternalism (interfering with a person's freedom for his or her own good) are also part of ethical decisions in civil commitment and compulsory treatment (Matusek & Wright, 2010).

Beneficence as a concept implies doing no harm and promoting the health and welfare of others (Beauchamp & Childress, 2001). However, when would it be reasonable to suggest beneficence implies taking over ones' decision making? To alter an eating disorder requires that the individual in therapy be intentionally distressed. This distress can be physical (weight restoration, rebound effects of purging or laxative abuse) or psychological (meaning inferred by weight gain, sense of loss of control when eating in a normal manner). When the distress is seen as too intense, the person in treatment may postponement treatment, refuse aspects of care, or stop treatment altogether. When these acts occur, beneficence would dictate that those decisions be respected by the care provider. However, following this ethical course will not further health and well-being and can lead to greater physical and psychological harm (Matusek & Wright, 2010). What then can a care provider do to navigate this thorny issue? One thought is to promote the idea that treatment must be risk-reducing with a primary goal of keeping the individual safe (Fedyszyn & Sullivan, 2007). Treatment must move from least restrictive (outpatient) to more structure and controlling (inpatient). Guidelines have been established by multiple psychiatric organizations regarding when to move to a more structured level of care (APA, 2006, National, G.A.U., 2017, Hilbert, Hoek, & Schmidt, 2017) and include for adults medical indications regarding weight < 85% of individually estimated healthy body weight; a heart rate < 40 bpm; blood pressure < 90/60 mm Hg; glucose < 60 mg/dL; potassium < 3 mEq/L; electrolyte imbalance; temperature < 97.0°F; dehydration; hepatic, renal, or cardiovascular organ compromise requiring acute treatment; and poorly controlled diabetes. For children and adolescents medical indications include weight < 85% of individually estimated healthy body weight or acute weight decline with food refusal; heart rate near 40 bpm; orthostatic hypotension (with an increase in pulse of > 20 bpm or a drop in blood pressure of > 10–20 mm Hg/minute from supine to standing; blood pressure < 80/50 mm Hg; hypokalemia, hypophosphatemia, or hypomagnesemia (APA, 2006). Other factors when considering hospitalization include suicidal intent with plan or other factors suggesting a high level of suicide risk; poor motivation to recover; and preoccupation with ego-syntonic or ego-dystonic maladaptive thoughts. Use of a hospital must considered when there is lack of cooperation with treatment or cooperation only in highly structured settings and a need for supervision during and after all meals and in bathrooms. Presence of additional stressors including the patient's ability to eat, significant psychosocial stressors or inadequate social supports, and weight near that at which medical instability occurred also warrants hospitalization (APA, 2006).

As can be seen, many things can influence hospitalization but from an ethical standpoint the patient can refuse the best guidelines for care if they are overwhelmed. At this point autonomy and beneficence collide with the care provider's need to promote health and well-being or prevent physical deterioration and possible death.

When this collision creates treatment refusal, beneficence in the form of civil commitment is the principal option (Fedyszyn & Sullivan, 2007). This view of civil commitment as promoting health and well-being is a balancing act for the care provider to find the maximum balance of benefit over harm (Beauchamp & Childress, 2001, Matusek & Wright, 2010).

When autonomy and beneficence are overridden, then the ethical principle of justice must be brought in to play. Justice means fairness, and in treatment settings it demands that the treated individual must have access to the best evidence-based care along with respect for the individual's dignity and the least restrictive measures to ensure a safe and positive outcome (Fedyszyn, Sullivan, Matusek, & Wright, 2010). While this is the ideal from an ethical standpoint, there is concern in the treatment of eating disorders that the "best care" may be granted to those who have the best insurance. In the case of civil commitment the individual can be "robbed" of their choice of care or treatment because that type of facility will not accept involuntary patients. Additionally, as commitment laws are specific to each state or province, the law does not travel from one area to another should the individual want the best evidence-based treatment. Justice as an ethical concept would suggest that treatment be available to the individual when they are hospitalized involuntarily. However, this is not always true when looking at treatment of an eating disorder (Andersen, 2007).

The ethical practice of justice means the right to be treated equally and the right to equal access to treatment. However, in actual practice, a number of different factors may influence actual access to treatment, for example, age, place of residence, social status, culture, disability, legal capacity, hospital budgets, and insurance coverage. Over the years a number of inpatient eating disorder programs have closed due to hospitals deeming those programs unprofitable (Hart, Granillo, Jorm, & Paxton, 2011, Vandereycken, 2003). So it is possible that dangerousness or grave disability could lead to civil commitment, but there would be no adequate treatment available. The demands of the principle of justice must apply at the bedside of individual patients but also systemically in the laws and policies of society that govern the access of a population to health care (Marques et al., 2011, Waller et al., 2009, Mond, Hay, Rodgers, & Owen, 2007).

Andersen (2008) suggests that social justice as an ethical perspective is on the lowest rung when focusing on patients with an eating disorder. The patient is the center of a broad social network of family members, caregivers, communities, governmental regulators, third-party payers, legislators, and judges. However, each aspect of that social network has its own self-serving goals, and, at times, its own counter-therapeutic practices.

Legislatures struggle with the concept of parity, but rarely do they offer equality of care for individuals with so-called mental disorders on the same level as medical conditions. Mental health is carved out for more limited health care benefits than "medical disorders," and eating disorders specifically have been the most ruthlessly reduced in coverage limitations. Psychiatric disorders often have a limited number of inpatient days with reduced aftercare visits and high copays. In contrast, "medical disorders" may have almost unlimited benefits. This leads to shorter inpatient treatments for patients with anorexia nervosa, despite evidence-based studies documenting that inpatient treatment short of an attempt at acute full remission leads to more relapses and more frequent rehospitalizations (Sebastian, & Hergenroeder, 2014). Rehospitalizations for patients with an eating disorder seem like standard operating procedure. Adequate care, which has longer lengths of stay, is considered an inappropriate and money-losing proposition, even though over the course of illness the latter costs less.

As Andersen (2007) points out, true social justice does not tolerate discrepancies in service based on race, gender, or sexual orientation. Excluding any population (such as males or individuals with bulimia nervosa) from inpatient or males from residential care programs represents an injustice, as does failure to reach out to diverse ethnic and racial communities. Data increasingly demonstrate that these groups have a high and increasing prevalence of eating disorders.

The health care training system may teach the importance of evidence-based treatment, but fail to provide training for psychiatrists in the most evidence-based psychotherapy for eating disorders, cognitive-behavioral therapy (CBT). Training in CBT has been largely abandoned in many hospital training programs. Unfortunately, too many programs neglect to provide residents with supervised experiences in the multiple therapeutic skills necessary for comprehensive treatment that include evidence-based psychotherapeutics (Marques et al., 2011, Waller et al., 2009, Mond et al., 2007).

Ethical use of social justice in the treatment of eating disorders demands access to quality care for all individuals. Advocacy for social justice includes comprehensive treatment programs with adequate reimbursement of care, funding of both clinical and transitional research studies for all eating disorders. There must be an end to discrimination in programs because of the type of insurance and regarding gender and increased screening for early diagnosis, and preventive intervention in demonstrated areas of effectiveness. Ethical social justice must combat the stigma surrounding eating disorders in particular that it is just a "bunch of spoiled young, privileged adolescents." States that currently do not admit severely ill anorexia nervosa patients for involuntary treatment even when clearly necessary in life-threatening cases need to remediate this deficit in view of evidence that selective involuntary admission and treatment can be lifesaving (Andersen, 2007).

Ethical considerations must be the cornerstone to excellent care for an individual with an eating disorder. These principles are paramount when considering civil commitment and involuntary treatment. Without an understanding of autonomy, beneficence, nonmaleficence, justice, and paternalism treatment becomes a shadow of respect for the patient. The use of ethical considerations must be part of every decision in treatment, especially when looking at overriding an individual's right to choose their care. Ethical issues must not be considered curiosities at the margin of treatment plans but should be incorporated into the mix of case discussions, morning rounds, treatment plans, and formal presentations.

References

American Psychiatric Association. (2006). Treatment of patients with eating disorders (3rd ed.). *American Journal of Psychiatry*, 163(7 Suppl), 4–54.

Andersen, A.E. (2007). Eating disorders and coercion. *American Journal of Psychiatry*, 164, 9–11.

Beauchamp, T.L., & Childress, J.F. (2001). *Principles of biomedical ethics*. Oxford: Oxford University Press.

Bratton, M. (2010). Anorexia, welfare, and the varieties of autonomy: Judicial rhetoric and the law in practice. *Philosophy, Psychiatry, & Psychology*, 17(2), 159–162.

Caplan, A.L. (2006). Ethical issues surrounding forced, mandated, or coerced treatment. *Journal of Substance Abuse Treatment*, 31(2), 117–120.

Craigie, J., Hope, T., Tan, J., Stewart, A., & McMillan, J. (2013). Agency, ambivalence and authenticity: The many ways in which anorexia nervosa can affect autonomy. *International Journal of Law in Context*, 9(1), 20–36.

Fedyszyn, I.E., & Sullivan, G.B. (2007). Ethical re-evaluation of contemporary treatments for anorexia nervosa: Is an aspirational stance possible in practice? *Australian Psychologist*, 42(3), 198–211.

Hart, L.M., Granillo, M.T., Jorm, A.F., & Paxton, S.J. (2011). Unmet need for treatment in the eating disorders: A systematic review of eating disorder specific treatment seeking among community cases. *Clinical Psychology Review*, 31(5), 727–735.

Hiday, V.A. (1996). Involuntary commitment as a psychiatric technology. *International Journal of Technology Assessment in Health Care*, 12, 585–603.

Hilbert, A., Hoek, H.W., & Schmidt, R. (2017). Evidence-based clinical guidelines for eating disorders: International comparison. *Current Opinion in Psychiatry*, 30(6), 423.

Kenney, D.W. (2012). Making Gandhi Ji eat: Dare we? Workshop presented at the 4th annual Eating Recovery Center Foundation Eating Disorders Conference, Denver, CO.

Marques, L., Alegria, M., Becker, A.E., Chen, C.N., Fang, A., Chosak, A., & Diniz, J.B. (2011). Comparative prevalence, correlates of impairment, and service utilization for eating disorders across US ethnic groups: Implications for reducing ethnic disparities in health care access for eating disorders. *International Journal of Eating Disorders*, 44(5), 412–420.

Matusek, J.A., & Wright, M.O.D. (2010). Ethical dilemmas in treating clients with eating disorders: A review and application of an integrative ethical decision-making model. *European Eating Disorders Review*, 18(6), 434–452.

Mond, J.M., Hay, P.J., Rodgers, B., & Owen, C. (2007). Health service utilization for eating disorders: Findings from a community-based study. *International Journal of Eating Disorders*, 40(5), 399–408.

National, G.A.U. (2017). *Eating disorders: Recognition and treatment.* National Guideline Alliance (UK). London: National Institute for Health and Care Excellence.

Sebastian, M.R., & Hergenroeder, A. (2014). Does rate of weight gain during hospitalization predict readmission in adolescents with eating disorders? *Journal of Adolescent Health*, 54(2), S78–S79.

Silber, T.J. (2011). Treatment of anorexia nervosa against the patient's will: Ethical considerations. *Adolescent Medicine—State of the Art Reviews*, 22(2), 283.

Swartz, M.S., Swanson, J.W., Wagner, H.R., Burns, B.J., Hiday, V.A., & Borum, R. (1999). Can involuntary outpatient commitment reduce hospital recidivism? Findings from a randomized trial with severely mentally ill individuals. *American Journal of Psychiatry*, 156, 1968–1975.

Tan, J.O., Hope, T., Stewart, A., & Fitzpatrick, R. (2003). Control and compulsory treatment in anorexia nervosa: The views of patients and parents. *International Journal of Law and Psychiatry*, 26(6), 627–645.

Tan, J., & Richards, L. (2015). Legal and ethical issues in the treatment of really sick patients with anorexia nervosa. In *Critical care for anorexia nervosa* (pp. 113–150). Berlin: Springer International.

Tansey, J. (2011). Ethical analysis: Civil commitment. Workshop presented at the 45th Association of Behavioral and Cognitive Therapy, Toronto, CA.

Vandereycken, W. (2003). The place of inpatient care in the treatment of anorexia nervosa: Questions to be answered. *International Journal of Eating Disorders*, 34(4), 409–422.

Waller, G., Schmidt, U., Treasure, J., Murray, K., Aleyna, J., Emanuelli, F., . . . Yeomans, M. (2009). Problems across care pathways in specialist adult eating disorder services. *Psychiatrist*, 33(1), 26–29.

5

Psychiatric Advanced Directives

Introduction

Every individual has the right to make the important decisions regarding their health care. Whether choosing to undergo a specific medical procedure, take certain medications, or receive life support, every individual exercises control over their treatment. The main process to assure the right to guide health care, especially when incapacitated, is the creation of a document that specifies the individual's wishes. These instructions are intended to inform loved ones and health providers of the patient's needs and concerns. These documents protect the individual from unwanted or harmful treatments and treatments that are ineffective. Control over decisions regarding medical care is globally supported with several international bodies supporting this perspective including the United Nations, European Union, Canada, Australia, New Zealand, and laws from all 50 United States (Bowers, 2014).

There are a variety of names such as living wills, proxy decision makers, and durable powers of attorney; advanced health care directives are used to communicate how medical care of a given individual must proceed. As a whole, these documents as commonly known as *advanced directives*. Simply defined, an advanced directive tells others what type of care the patient would like if or when they become unable to make or convey their decisions.

Advantages of Advanced Directives

An advanced directive clearly states the individual's wishes and attitudes on all medical interventions and future care decisions. If a patient becomes incapacitated, an advanced directive informs the health care provider what specific care is desired and what is not. Family and friends who are aware of the advanced directive can make treatment decisions that are informed by the patient's personal requests. An advanced directive offers guidance to health care providers to focus on the individual's wishes when confronted with difficult decisions. Similarly, this type of document creates opportunities for family and health providers to discuss palliative care, hospice, and end of life issues. Advanced directives address treatments to be used or rejected, especially those which would be seen as uncomfortable, having undesirable side effects, and that would fail to improve quality of life (Olsen, 2017, Westmoreland & Mehler, 2017).

There are distinct limitations to advanced directives. These documents cannot mandate anything considered illegal by the local, state, or national justice system. This type of document could not create interventions outside of current medical procedure or limit access to a person's basic needs such as food, water, or activities of daily living. Advanced directives have three general types. A living will states the individual's wishes regarding future health care, whether in general terms or relating only to specific situations and circumstances. A health care proxy/durable power of attorney appoints another person to act on their behalf regarding future health care decisions if they become incapacitated. The third type of advanced directive is a medical directive, which is a request that is a part of the individual's medical record. An example would be a do not resuscitate (DNR) order (Olsen, 2017, Westmoreland & Mehler, 2017).

General Points

Advanced directives offer opportunities for friends, family, and health care professionals to have ongoing discussions to determine the patient's wants and needs. Although this collaboration regarding the individual's wishes is vital for future health care, an advanced directive can only reflect a person's wishes at the time at which it was created. The person writing the advanced directive must be considered capable or competent to make such life-sustaining or life-ending determinations. Generally, advanced directives do not need to be complicated and in many states, provinces, or countries, a handwritten document stating one's wishes is enough. However, some countries, provinces, and states have specific forms that need to be completed in order for the directive to be recognized legally (Olsen, 2017, Westmoreland & Mehler, 2017).

Advance Directives for Mental Health Treatment

What Is a Psychiatric Advance Directive?

A psychiatric advance directive (PAD) is similar in many respects to a medical advanced directives but is specific to mental health care. Broadly, a PAD is a legal document written by a currently competent person who lives with a mental illness. This legal document allows a person to give instructions for future mental health treatment or appoint a person to make future decisions about mental health treatment. A PAD prepares the patient who, in the midst of a mental health crisis, cannot make decisions about his or her care. The document is helpful during an acute stage or exacerbation of a long-standing illness to assist the patient in communicating decisions about his/her treatment. A PAD conveys treatment preferences, or names of individuals to make treatment decisions, when the patient cannot (Slade, 2017, Castillo, Castillo, Ramon, & Ramon, 2017, Zelle, Kempf, & Bonnie, 2015).

Two general versions of a psychiatric advance directive can be created. An instructive PAD provides instructions about specific mental health treatment and includes desired options to avoid or minimize hospitalization. The PAD can identify preferred stress-relieving activities; preferred or problematic medications; and identify preferences regarding the use of certain treatments, interventions, emergency contacts, and lists of activities known to worsen symptoms like electroconvulsive therapy (APA, 2006).

A proxy PAD designates individuals who make treatment decisions when the patient is unable to do so. The designated individual is established as a person with treatment power of attorney or decision-making authority. Use of this preference means the individual must select an agent who understands the role and responsibilities, as well as the mental health system. The individual with a power of attorney must make decisions that reflect what the patient would prefer. The individual with power of attorney is expected to make decisions that will reflect the best interest of the patient including medication preferences, inpatient treatment, and that changes in wellness can occur (Slade, 2017, Castillo et al., 2017, Zelle et al., 2015).

The National Resource Center on Psychiatric Advance Directives (2015) notes two main reasons to create a psychiatric advance directive: (1) to make possible you are treated according to your wishes and (2) to facilitate a more informed and open dialogue with your treatment provider. The Council on Psychiatry and Law of the American Psychiatric Association also identifies several reasons to create PAD (APA, May 2009). Creation of a PAD can enhance the collaborative process and communication between the psychiatrist and patient. A PAD can also empower patients to engage directly in their treatment. The collaborative process of creating a PAD between the patient and psychiatrist strengthens the therapeutic alliance and improves overall clinical outcomes. A PAD can lead to greater patient satisfaction and a more positive attitude toward treatment providers. PADs may help the patient feel in control over his or her treatment.

Many states, provinces, and countries have enacted laws allowing advance directives for general medical purposes; however, these advanced directive laws may or may not apply to psychiatric illnesses. In the United States, 25 states have enacted psychiatric-specific advance directives (Arizona, Hawaii, Indiana, Idaho, Illinois, Kentucky, Louisiana, Maine, Maryland, Michigan, Minnesota, Montana, New Jersey, New Mexico, North Carolina, Oregon, Ohio, Oklahoma, Pennsylvania, South Dakota, Tennessee, Texas, Utah, Washington, and Wyoming). These laws are intended to empower individuals with mental illnesses, provided they are competent to express their preferences for the acceptance or refusal of psychiatric treatment just as they are allowed to accept or refuse treatment for physical illness (Zelle et al., 2015).

While most laws presume that a person is competent when he or she drafts advance directives, some jurisdictions apply stricter standards when it comes to utilizing them in mental health care decisions. States, provinces, and countries vary in their requirements for the determination of competence. In some areas, for example, judges must make competence, or legal capacity, decisions before the advance directive can be followed. Incapacity means the individual lacks sufficient understanding or ability to make and communicate mental health treatment decisions. However, the legal definition of incapacity varies from state to state and province to province, and some states or provinces do not define incapacity. Usually, incapacity is determined by a physician or eligible psychologist, but in some areas it must be determined by a judge or magistrate. Competence and capacity become important in the creation and implementation of a psychiatric advanced directive.

A PAD is an important tool for the prevention of unwanted treatment while maintaining a patient's power over their mental health care. A PAD creates very explicit preferences regarding type and place of care. Specifically it can state the desired treatments including which medications to be prescribed. More important, a PAD would specify medicines or treatments that would be acceptable. Unfortunately, psychiatric advance directives are not understood or often ignored especially for individuals with reoccurring and debilitating mental health issues. An additional advantage of a PAD is cooperation between the patient's mental health care representative, family, friends, and mental health care professionals to work as a team to support the wishes and desires of patient. With this advantage in mind, it is very important that the patient must be diligent in their choice of who will speak for them when the PAD is implemented (Zelle et al., 2015).

Psychiatric Advanced Directives

There are circumstances when a PAD would not be recognized. Primary is the application of civil commitment. Civil commitment and involuntary treatment takes priority over the stipulation of psychiatric advanced directive. Additionally, a PAD can be overridden when it conflicts with "generally accepted community practice standards," the treatments requested are not feasible or available, or when it conflicts with emergency treatment. However, preferences regarding medication and other aspects of treatment while hospitalized should be followed even when involuntarily committed (Bowers, 2014).

As an alternative to civil commitment or a follow-up after the commitment has ended, a PAD can help minimize many of the ambiguities commonly associated with mental health crises (Sarin, 2012, Srebnik, 2005). Psychiatric advanced directives are legal documents that allow competent individuals, through advance instructions and/or designation of a health care agent, to declare preferences for future mental health treatment. With a more long-term or chronic disorder such as anorexia nervosa, a PAD can be potentially helpful for the following reasons: (1) it can empower consumers to assume control over treatment decisions; (2) it can enhance communications about treatment preferences between consumers, families, and treatment providers; (3) it may facilitate appropriate and timely interventions before situations deteriorate to emergency status; and (4) it may lead to reductions in adversarial court proceedings over involuntary psychiatric treatment (Sarin, 2012, Srebnik, 2005, Swanson, Van McCrary, Swartz, Elbogen, & Van Doren, 2006).

Most state statutes presume that people are competent at the time they draft advance directives. These laws generally require the directive to be signed by two adult witnesses who attest to the person's capacity at the time the instrument is drafted. More difficult questions arise over determining capacity at the time advance directives are used for health care decisions. In some states, provinces, or countries a judge must make capacity determinations. Another controversial issue concerns the potential use of PAD to refuse all treatment. All states that authorize PAD, except Maine, specify that individuals or patients may use these directives to consent or refuse psychiatric treatment unless the patient is a danger to self or others or by not obtaining assistance they create grave disability (Sarin, 2012, Srebnik, 2005)

An unresolved question concerns revocation of PAD. These laws establish the right of persons with mental illnesses to write directives, when competent, indicating their wishes concerning acceptance or refusal of psychiatric treatment. Clearly, an individual may revoke a PAD when competent. While PADs are quite promising for empowering consumers to more actively participate in their treatment, there are legitimate concerns about these instruments and the possibility of abuse. One of the thorniest issues concerns determinations of legal capacity or competence. Questions about capacity arise at two different points in the process. First, individuals or patients must be competent at the time they draft a PAD for these documents to be valid. Second, a PAD may be used for psychiatric decisions only when the individual or patient is not competent to make these decisions by himself or herself. A more difficult question arises when an individual tries to revoke their PAD while actively symptomatic and in need of treatment. The insertion of a so-called Ulysses clause in an advance directive could effectively avoid this dilemma (Sarin, 2012).

This name originated from the Greek hero, Ulysses, who knew that the song of the beautiful Sirens was so powerful that he would be compelled to sail his ship toward the rocks thereby destroying it. He ordered his men to bind him to the mast of the ship and to keep sailing straight, no matter how strongly he argued to the contrary. A Ulysses clause instructs treatment providers about specific treatment preferences, and explains that any statements made refusing treatment during periods of incapacity should be ignored (Sarin, 2012, Srebnik, 2005).

How Psychiatric Advanced Directives Might Work With Treating Eating Disorders

If a psychiatric advanced directive was developed for an individual with an eating disorder, what might be the general goals? One focus would be on treatment preferences. This could include decisions when to make a change from an outpatient level of care to a more intense treatment setting. An example would be an individual who is working on weight restoration plateaus or begins a downward slide. A written PAD could suggest very specific interventions such as admission to an intensive outpatient program, partial hospital program or residential treatment center. The objective would be to intervene prior to the need for inpatient care.

During the early stages of treatment the development of specific interventions could be agreed upon if there is no significant progress. Along those same lines, a psychiatric advanced directive could be part of discharge planning after inpatient care. Collaborative development of a written PAD could engage the patient, significant others, or family members and the health care provider into a better understanding of the needs of the patient. In a similar manner a PAD could establish a threshold for hospitalization that could shorten length of stay if the individual's weight or physical or psychological condition became dangerous.

Much of what can transpire with a PAD is based on the capacity of the person who writes the directive. If there is a concern about capacity, the PAD may be dismissed. However, writing this type of directive early in treatment and/or at a transition point of care (inpatient to a partial hospital program) could potentially alter the course of treatment and reduce repeated hospitalization, which has been correlated to poorer outcomes in the treatment of eating disorders (Zelle et al., 2015). Although untested, this approach may have merits across all ages and especially with those patients with severe and enduring eating disorders (Zelle et al., 2015).

Severe and Enduring Eating Disorders (SEED)

The concepts of a severe and enduring eating disorder (SEED; Robinson, Kukucska, Guidetti, & Leavey, 2015) and severe enduring anorexia nervosa (Touyz & Strober, 2016) are areas where a PAD could offer direct benefit. Robinson (Robinson et al., 2015) identifies these individuals with a long-term and complex presentation of anorexia nervosa which limits or inhibits medical, social, occupational, and familial well-being. He suggests the establishment of a multidisciplinary treatment team with a collaborative behavioral contract that is flexible and avoids "dehumanizing, rigidly monitored control battles around eating behavior." This collaborative behavioral contract could be a PAD. Following Robinson's model, a PAD would include avoidance of overly controlled behavioral plans about weight restoration and a focus on basic requirements regarding medical monitoring. Along with medical monitoring, when there is a shift to outpatient care there would be a need for a clear criteria for hospitalization. If new empirically supported treatments are developed, they would need to discuss those particular psychotherapeutic or pharmacological interventions.

Robinson's ideas are consistent with Strober's (2004) suggestions regarding the treatment of the long-term individual with an eating disorder. Based on Strober, a PAD would emphasize unambiguous assurance that weight gain is not the objective of treatment. The maintenance of a positive quality of life with increased social activity would be the driving principle to further prevent psychological invalidation and isolation. To ensure this outcome the PAD would require regular physical examinations with a psychologically informed collaborating physician to help guide treatment decisions. Family and significant other involvement would be written into the psychiatric advanced directive, including education about the disorder in order to provide solace and to discourage disparagement and anger toward the patient. The ideas established by Robinson and Strober fit easily into a PAD.

Other authors have developed approaches to this population that also fit into a PAD paradigm. Kaplan (Kaplan & Strasburg, 2009, Kaplan & Strasburg, 2009) reports on the use of Assertive Community Treatment (ACTS) which provides client-centered, community-based interventions for clients with serious and enduring anorexia nervosa. The ideas in this approach work to maintain the individual out of a hospital level of care and relies on a client-centered approach to maintain autonomy rather than a symptoms focused approach that favors paternalism. Again, the primary focus of treatment is quality of life rather than changing weight or eating behavior. With a PAD the written plan would emphasize assessment of physical status that might disrupt quality of life while remaining alert for psychological change toward recovery. Broad goals that could be part of a written PAD are engagement in vocational counseling, housing support, enhanced social supports, and facilitating medical stabilization and reducing duration of hospitalization when needed, thereby maintaining the individual's autonomy.

Williams, Dobney, and Geller (2010) have promoted the Community Outreach Partnership Program (COPP) as a means to working with more severely ill individuals with eating disorders. Their primary goals are quality of life and increasing independence rather than decreasing symptoms. This integrated program fits well into a psychiatric advanced directive. The program includes staff from a hospital-based eating disorder program and a community-based mental health rehabilitation team. All clinical contact with the patient takes place in the community (e.g., home, other community agencies) with an emphasis on the importance of environmental resources and the development of a broad-based community of individuals and institutions that support the patient's well-being. Williams et al. identify "nonnegotiables" that refer to essential agreements the patient must make in order to be seen by the COPP team (e.g., attendance at medical appointments) which fit into the broad concept of a PAD.

Yager (2007) also wrote of a framework and developed recommendations about working with severe and enduring eating disordered patients. Primary to this approach is maintaining individual autonomy by establishing a connection with the patient and establish consistent goals that avoid counterproductive battles over control of treatment. The goals and plans can take a written form consistent with a psychiatric advanced directive. The plan also works to engage the patient's family and significant others to play a pivotal role in what treatment would be if there would be a deterioration in the patient's physical or mental status. Along with patient and family involvement, a multidisciplinary treatment team would develop a collaborative behavioral contract that is flexible and avoids battles around eating behavior. As part of this plan, it is very important to maintain the basic requirements regarding medical monitoring and a written criteria for hospitalization. Equally important is avoidance of expensive, time-consuming treatments that have been repeatedly ineffective or instill unfounded hope. A psychiatric advanced directive would also develop when to consider legal procedures (civil commitment) only in life-threatening situations. This approach emphasizes the application of humanistic treatment principles that respect the patient's self-determination and autonomy, but also mandates clinicians to impose interventions in potentially harmful circumstances.

A PAD can be used to determine treatment when an individual is either hospitalized or incapacitated. A PAD could strongly suggest that the hospital-based treatment team create a highly individualized plan focusing on maintenance goals rather than emphasizing active symptom change. Hospital-based programs with a primary focus on weight restoration and psychotherapy that develop a plan addressing overall health and quality of life will be more beneficial. The PAD may require modifications in group therapies and other components of treatment in which patients interact (Robinson et al., 2015).

Another area in which a PAD would work is to request those with severe and enduring anorexia nervosa to engage in short-term hospitalizations on medical units. Although not generally the first line of treatment, there are programs that specifically treat individual on medical units (Gaudiani, Sabel, Mascolo, & Mehler, 2012).

Hospital units that accept eating disorder patients of this severity for medical stabilization should have staff who are well trained in eating disorders and understand more intense cases without the goal and expectations for full recovery. If medical units are used, once medical stabilization is reached, these patients should be transferred to an eating disorder unit and offered psychiatric and nutritional interventions, and stepped down to outpatient care. Robinson et al. (2015) suggests that with proper supervision, most medical complications can be managed in an inpatient eating disorder treatment setting, so treatment strictly on a medical unit may be overridden in a PAD.

A PAD could make an effective tool in the treatment of eating disorders creating an alternative to civil commitment. Hay, Touyz, and Sud (2012) support moving beyond the core aspects of inpatient treatment (primarily weight restoration) and examine efficacy and effectiveness in minimizing harm and reducing personal and social costs of chronic illness. When writing a psychiatric advanced directive, treatment can be established using the ideas of Strober and others (Hay et al., 2012, Robinson et al., 2015, Yager, 2007) who advocate and emphasize therapeutic alliance and flexible goals. Also treatment like CBT modified for anorexia nervosa, cognitive remediation therapy with emotion skills training, the Maudsley Model for Treatment of Adults with Anorexia Nervosa, the Community Outreach Partnership Program, and Specialist Supportive Clinical Management must be considered when developing a PAD. Of paramount importance is to address the needs and desires of individuals while maintaining treatment that moves from a focus on dangerousness to grave disability and emphasizes the best quality of life possible (Hay et al., 2012).

The use of PAD is in its infancy. There are more unresolved questions than answers about these instruments. Ongoing research projects and pending court decisions will provide more comprehensive information in the future. A parallel study with Huntington's disease has been suggested as template for ED (Bisson, Hampton, Rosser, & Holm, 2009). Having easy-to-follow instructions, consistent verbal and written information helped completers of PAD feel empowered by the process (Henderson et al., 2004). Psychiatric advanced directives may help patients with ED face the seriousness of their condition without diminishing their self-esteem (Sheehan, 2009, Thiels & Curtice, 2009). Until then, PAD must be strongly considered as a way to empower consumers to take an active role in their own treatment, and as a way to avoid damaging, divisive conflicts over treatment and medication issues.

Psychiatric Advanced Directives: Ethical Considerations

When one looks to help individuals maintain autonomy in their psychiatric health care choice, a PAD could be a step forward. Clear decision making about how others attend to those stated needs could reduce or perhaps prevent civil commitment. Schwartz and Mack (2004) suggests that a PAD could allow a greater sense of autonomy by the individual to help engage health care workers in treatment and improve the process of care during a crisis. If the PAD can maintain autonomy while a person is in crisis, then it does help the individual attain the care they desire as long as it meets the current medical standard of care. However, a PAD can lack the strength or legal mechanism to assure that the individual's wishes occurred or were written during a period of competence (Swartz & Mack, 2004, Swartz, Swanson, & Elbogen, 2004).

Given a desire to maintain control over one's care (autonomy), assisting an individual to express those needs is paramount, especially if the individual wants to prevent involuntary treatment. The plans developed in a PAD have at potential to help guide hard treatment decisions during times of crisis and are intended help caregivers honor the wishes of the individual and help maintain their autonomy and self-determination. However, as Swanson et al. (2006) point out, a PAD can be overridden by civil commitment laws. It is important to make all parties involved the PAD aware of this limitation.

Swanson et al. (2006) summarize three situations in which a PAD can be overridden: first, when the PAD does not reasonably reflect what the individual wants; second, when the PAD conflicts with what is known to be the personal interests of the individual; and third, when the interest of other persons' warrant an override such as safety of those who could not protect themselves. These situations could occur when there is severe and persistent mental illness.

Of primary focus in a severe emotional disorder are events that create a danger to self or others. There is no legal mechanism that will enforce a patient's right to refuse all treatment during a time when the individual is in a danger to self or others. To contest or reduce the potential for override, it is suggested that a highly specific PAD be developed. In addition, Swanson et al. (2006) indicate that a PAD may be unethical as it can be viewed as a document that favors the individual's prior self (e.g. competent) rather than the individual's current self. Danger to self or others trumps any PAD or refusal of treatment. Also, if the PAD infers there is a conflict between the individual's personal choice (involuntary treatment, nutritional rehabilitation) and their safety, then the PAD could be morally and legally challenged (Kenney, 2012, Tansey, 2011).

Appelbaum (2006) presents a different argument. His view is that even when there is involuntary treatment, if the individual has a preference between equally reasonable treatment choices, these preferences should be respected. If there is a specific rejection of a treatment (type of nutritional rehabilitation), then that preference should be respected unless there is no other viable treatments available. He notes that development of a PAD often implies the individual who completes PAD has a treatable condition, with the probability of substantial symptomatic improvement and marked increase in functioning. Helping individuals maintain autonomy via PAD could reduce long-term hospitalization. However, he does suggest, allowing individuals to decline treatment through PADs especially when there is no reason improve their emotional condition imposes a burden to society of indefinite care for persons with serious mental disorders. Although it may promote autonomy for the individual, there must be exceptions that focus on the greater good of the community or family.

An important ethical aspect of treatment is informed consent. Writing a PAD represents evidence of informed consent for future treatment to be implemented later when capacity is compromised (Easter, Swanson, Robertson, Moser, & Swartz, 2017). A psychiatric advanced directive, especially when it indicates refusal of treatment, is simply a valid way for a person to indicate an objection to certain interventions. However, there must be confirmation that the individual who created the PAD had the capacity to make a reasoned choice of care. Even though the PAD represents an individual's autonomy when competent refusing or limiting treatment might indicate to the caregiver or proxy decision maker how the disorder can overwhelm the individual's ability to make beneficial decisions (lack of autonomy). Ethically, refusal of or limitations to interventions in a PAD can and must be overridden especially when those requests are for non-standard care (Easter et al., 2017).

There are times when caregivers may not readily accept the validity of the individuals' preferences for psychiatric treatment. This is especially true when there is treatment refusal or limitations on type of treatment. Also, validity can be challenged when the patient's choice of interventions does not meet the current medical standard of care. An ethical mental health care provider who wants to preserve autonomy must recognize that the intent of the PAD is to be proactive (Easter et al., 2017). The responsibility of the mental health provider with the individual, family, and or proxy decision maker documents the personal preferences of the patient in ways that will increase the likelihood that PADs will be understood and honored. Collaboration can foster trust and engagement, and promote therapeutic alliances between patients and their mental health care providers, which can represent a form of informed consent (Easter et al., 2017). A caveat has been presented by Elbogen, Van Dorn, Swanson, Swartz, and Monahan, (2006), pointing out that although the law presumes that people are competent to complete PADs, because mental illness often involves fluctuating decisional capacity, the patient's ability to write a PAD may be questioned. From a practical standpoint, clinicians may raise the issue of competence to complete a PAD when a patient documents a refusal of standard treatment. If patients show no such impairments at the time, it may still be advisable for patients to explicitly state in the PAD their reasons for a treatment refusal (Elbogen et al., 2006).

Conclusion

In a qualitative analysis of patients' views of psychiatric advance directives, participants consistently viewed them as a positive tool to promote autonomy with the potential to facilitate stronger patient-provider relationships. However, they expressed concerns about limited knowledge among service providers and difficulties communicating the directives to inpatient staff. Studies also suggest that when offered greater self-determination individuals with mental illness have a higher quality of life and better community integration. Van Dorn et al., (2010) states that the use of psychiatric advanced directives improve treatment outcomes especially in the area of coercive interventions like involuntary commitment. Perhaps it is time to formally look at the use of PAD as part of the overall treatment of eating disorders and not just at a time when the individual may be incapacitated.

References

American Psychiatric Association. (2006). Treatment of patients with eating disorders (3rd ed.). *American Journal of Psychiatry*, 163(7 Suppl), 4–54.

Appelbaum, P.S. (2006). History of civil commitment and related reforms in the United States: Lessons for today. *Developments in Mental Health Law*, 25, 13.

Bisson, J.I., Hampton, V., Rosser, A., & Holm, S. (2009). Developing a care pathway for advance decisions and powers of attorney: qualitative study. *British Journal of Psychiatry*, 194(1), 55–61.

Bowers, W.A. (2014). Civil commitment in the treatment of eating disorders and substance abuse: Empirical status and ethical considerations. In *Eating disorders, addictions and substance use disorders* (pp. 649–664). Berlin: Springer.

Castillo, H., Castillo, H., Ramon, S., & Ramon, S. (2017). "Work with me": Service users' perspectives on shared decision making in mental health. *Mental Health Review Journal*, 22(3), 166–178.

Council on Psychiatry and Law Psychiatric: Advance Directives (2009). Washington, DC: American Psychiatric Association.

Easter, M.M., Swanson, J.W., Robertson, A.G., Moser, L.L., & Swartz, M.S. (2017). Facilitation of psychiatric advance directives by peers and clinicians on assertive community treatment teams. *Psychiatric Services*, 68(7), 717–723.

Elbogen, E.B., Van Dorn, R.A., Swanson, J.W., Swartz, M.S., & Monahan, J. (2006). Treatment engagement and violence risk in mental disorders. *British Journal of Psychiatry*, 189(4), 354–360.

Gaudiani, J.L., Sabel, A.L., Mascolo, M., & Mehler, P.S. (2012). Severe anorexia nervosa: outcomes from a medical stabilization unit. *International Journal of Eating Disorders*, 45(1), 85–92.

Hay, P.J., Touyz, S., & Sud, R. (2012). Treatment for severe and enduring anorexia nervosa: a review. *Australian & New Zealand Journal of Psychiatry*, 46(12), 1136–1144.

Henderson, C., Flood, C., Leese, M., Thornicroft, G., Sutherby, K., & Szmukler, G. (2004). Effect of joint crisis plans on use of compulsory treatment in psychiatry: Single blind randomised controlled trial. *British Medical Journal*, 329, 136–138.

Kaplan, A.S., & Strasburg, K. (2009). Chronic eating disorders: a different approach to treatment resistance. *Psychiatric Times*, 26(8), 31–31.

Kaye, W. (2009). Eating disorders: Hope despite mortal risk. *American Journal of Psychiatry*, 166, 1309–1311.

Kenney, D.W. (2012). *Making Gandhi Ji eat: Dare we?* Workshop presented at the 4th annual Eating Recovery Center Foundation Eating Disorders Conference, Denver, CO.

Olsen, D.P. (2017). Increasing the use of psychiatric advance directives. *Nursing Ethics*, 24(3) 265–267.

Robinson, P.H., Kukucska, R., Guidetti, G., & Leavey, G. (2015). Severe and enduring anorexia nervosa (SEED-AN): A qualitative study of patients with 20+ years of anorexia nervosa. *European Eating Disorders Review*, 23(4), 318–326.

Sarin, A. (2012). On psychiatric wills and the Ulysses clause: The advance directive in psychiatry. *Indian Journal of Psychiatry*, 54, 206.

Schwartz, H.I., & Mack, D.M. (2003). Informed consent and competency. In R. Rosner (Ed.), *Principles and practice of forensic psychiatry* (pp. 97–106). New York: Taylor & Francis.

Sheehan, K.A., & Burns, T. (2011). Perceived coercion and the therapeutic relationship: a neglected association? *Psychiatric Services*, 62(5), 471–476.

Slade, M. (2017). Implementing shared decision making in routine mental health care. *World Psychiatry*, 16(2), 146–153.

Srebnik, D.S., Rutherford, L.T., Peto, T., Russo, J., Zick, E., Jaffe, C., & Holtzheimer, P. (2005). The content and clinical utility of psychiatric advance directives. *Psychiatric Services*, 56, 592–598.

Strober, M. (2004). Managing the chronic, treatment-resistant patient with anorexia nervosa. *International Journal of Eating Disorders*, 36(3), 245–255.

Swanson, J.W., Van McCrary, S., Swartz, M.S., Elbogen, E.B., & Van Dorn, R.A. (2006). Superseding psychiatric advance directives:

Ethical and legal considerations. *Journal of the American Academy of Psychiatry and the Law Online*, 34, 385–394.

Swartz, M.S., Swanson, J.W., & Elbogen, E.B. (2004). Psychiatric advance directives: Practical, legal, and ethical issues. *Journal of Forensic Psychology Practice*, 4(4), 97–107.

Tansey, J. (2011). *Ethical analysis: Civil commitment.* Workshop presented at the 45th Association of Behavioral and Cognitive Therapy, Toronto, CA.

Thiels, C., & Curtice, M.J. (2009). Forced treatment of anorexic patients: Part 2. *Current Opinion in Psychiatry*, 22, 497–500.

Touyz, S., & Strober, M. (2016). Managing the patient with severe and enduring anorexia nervosa. In S. Touyz, D. Le Grange, H. Lacey, & P. Hay (Eds.), *Managing severe and enduring anorexia nervosa: A clinician's guide* (pp. 95–111). New York: Routledge.

Treatment Advocacy Center. (2013, January). State standards for assisted treatment: Civil commitment criteria for inpatient and outpatient psychiatric treatment. Retrieved from www.treat mentadvocacycenter.org

Van Dorn, R.A., Scheyett, A., Swanson, J.W., & Swartz, M.S. (2010). Psychiatric advance directives and social workers: an integrative review. *Social Work*, 55(2), 157–167.

Westmoreland, P., & Mehler, P.S. (2017). Ethical principles. In P.S. Mehler & A.E. Andersen (Eds.), *Eating disorders: A guide to medical care and complications* (pp. 278–309). Baltimore, MD: Johns Hopkins Press.

Williams, K.D., Dobney, T., & Geller, J. (2010). Setting the eating disorder aside: An alternative model of care. *European Eating Disorders Review*, 18(2), 90–96.

Yager, J. (2007). Management of patients with chronic, intractable eating disorders. *Clinical manual of eating disorders* (pp. 407–439). Washington, DC: American Psychiatric.

Yager, J., Carney, T., & Touyz, S. (2016). Is involuntary (compulsory) treatment ever justified in patients with SE-AN: An international perspective. In S. Touyz, D. LeGrange, H. Lacey, & P. Hay

(Eds.), *Managing severe and enduring anorexia nervosa: A clinician's guide* (pp. 185–201). Abingdon: Routledge.

Zelle, H., Kemp, K., & Bonnie, R.J. (2015). Advance directives in mental health care: evidence, challenges and promise. *World Psychiatry*, 14(3), 278–280.

6

Compassionate Use of Civil Commitment

What is compassion? Compassion, according to Merriam-Webster, is the sympathetic consciousness of others' distress together with a desire to alleviate it. Compassion is a feeling state that arises when you are confronted with another's suffering and feel motivated to relieve that suffering. Compassion is when those feelings and thoughts are accompanied by a strong desire to alleviate the suffering. The treatment of eating disorders ethically and practically must be compassionate (Russell, 2001, Andersen, 2008). Compassion for the individual who because of a disabling illness has lost their capacity to make decisions that empowers them to a full and valued life (Tan & Richards, 2015, Carney, 2014). Compassion for the individual who by virtue of their illness has lost how to assess their self-worth based on something other than weight, shape, size and appearance (Fairburn, 2008). Compassion for the individual who based on their disorder put themselves in harm's way for physical and psychological damage that could become lifelong and potentially irreversible (Mehler & Andersen, 2017). Compassion for those individuals who risk death at a higher rate than other emotional disorders. Compassion for those individuals who view themselves through a prism that values thinness and control as their sole identity and fear any alteration of that worldview as an assault on their person (Tan & Richards, 2015, Carney, 2014). Compassion is as fundamental as autonomy, beneficence, non-maleficence, and justice when treating individuals with an eating disorder. But compassion also can run contrary to these ethical principles when treatment is refused or capacity to make reasoned or rational decisions is overridden by an eating disorder. How then do clinicians, family members, or significant others assist the individual with an eating disorder in a compassionate manner? How do you balance autonomy and the right to refuse treatment with the dire need to assist in weight restoration, interfere with binge and purge behavior, and return to normal health? The answer is to establish serious interventions that include adequate and consistent nutrition and improve the overall physical and psychological health and quality of life. Engage in interventions that decrease the likelihood of the disorder moving from intensely interfering in one's life to chronic morbidity and significant mortality. Compassion dictates that these treatments must be implemented even when they are refused.

Options have been suggested to address noncompliance and treatment refusal. Clinicians have options including altering the treatment contract away from addressing the eating disorder and focusing on overall issues such as self-esteem (Strober, 2006). Another approach is to discuss factors that make it hard for the therapist and individual to accept the treatment "nonnegotiables" such as increasing caloric intake, reduction of purging, or reduction and/or short-term elimination of exercise, diuretics, and laxatives. A clinician can present an "ultimatum" about treatment, and if the individual is not willing to able to engage in change then treatment can be suspended until the individual is ready (Goldner, Birmingham, & Smye, 1997). All of the above can be and most likely have been implemented, especially on an outpatient basis, in the treatment of an eating disorder. Whether to end therapy is beyond the scope of this chapter, but moving from the central tenet that change for a person with an eating disorder must have weight restoration (anorexia nervosa) reduction and cessation of binge and purge behavior (broadly, vomiting, laxative use and so on) places the clinician in a dilemma of how to best intervene especially when the outcome of nonintervention may be irreversible physical and psychological problems. It is in this battleground that compassion for the future of the individual (the desire to relieve suffering and assist with change) run into the autonomy to make one's own decisions about their life. It is also a moment where decisions about when and how to intervene are hardest. It is a juncture that compassion directs the clinician toward overriding autonomy by being aware that the behavior of the individual does not come from free choice but are resultant from a deadly disruptive disease (Goldner, 1989). When this occurs, civil commitment must be considered in a congruent and responsible manner, sharing with the individual the nature and course of the illness and ultimate consequences of the illness if no change were to occur (Dresser, 1984a, 1984b).

How does civil commitment become compassionate? By concentrating on preserving life. It is consensus that civil commitment and involuntary treatment are paramount when an individual who has an eating disorder is in medical jeopardy (Yager, Carney, & Touyz, 2016, Elzakkers, Danner, Hoek, Schmidt, & van Elburg, 2014). Whether employed as a last resort when other treatments have failed or implemented during inpatient treatment when a desire to discharge would contribute to risk of medical instability and place the individual in grave danger, compassion demands action. Civil commitment is the action that can stop the deteriorating effects of the illness while enhancing the potential of improvement that will lead to a return to outpatient care.

This move to undermine autonomy can be supported by an argument that those who refuse treatment may not have capacity to make good decisions or the illness deprives the person of the ability to make autonomous decisions (Bowers, 2014). Silber (2011) has conjected that autonomy can be compromised by a debilitating illness, and when this occurs there is a need to override autonomy with justified paternalism. Caplan (2006) has put forth the argument that respect for self-determination sometimes requires mandatory treatment as a way to create or enable autonomy. The premise is that people who lack capacity are not self-determined or autonomous because they are caught up in their illness. If this is indeed true, then it may be possible to justify civil commitment and compulsory treatment in order to return autonomy to the affected individual. Caplan (2006) also advances the idea that the illness itself can be a form of coercion. Physiological and psychological symptoms such as a drive for thinness, purging, and anxiety about weight gain are powerful motivators to continue behavior. Civil commitment offers an opportunity to facilitate change and increase an individual's autonomy and ability to maintain health. Maintaining health and the ability to make good choices about their actions in the long run would be the compassionate and ethical thing to do (Caplan, 2006).

Another modest support for civil commitment as a compassionate approach comes from individuals who develop an eating disorder. The scant literature (Tan, Hope, Stewart, & Patrick, 2003, Tan, Stewart, Fitzpatrick, & Hope, 2010) on the attitudes of individuals with an eating disorder found that although reluctant to accept civil commitment there was a grudging acknowledgment of the need for care. Specifically, civil commitment was appropriate because no one should die because of an eating disorder (Tan et al., 2003, Tan et al., 2010). Ancillary to this view was the individual's concept that being at an extremely low weight limited their capacity for decision making and supported decision making was appropriate. Tan et al. (2003) indicate that, at times, the individual cannot make a good choice even if that is their desire and that being "coerced" might be what was "wanted" to help make a choice for change and treatment.

One discussion about civil commitment centers on whether this action would inhibit the therapeutic relationship (Sheehan, 2009, Sheehan & Burns, 2011). Empirical data are lacking, with most references being anecdotal (Werth, Wright, Archambault, & Bardash, 2003). The implication is that civil commitment and violating an individual's autonomy is counterproductive in short-term and long-term treatment (Dresser, 1984a, Dresser 1984b). This is balanced by others who feel that the use of civil commitment is, after the fact, seen as an important step toward the goal of change and overcoming an eating disorder (Andersen, Bowers, & Evans, 1997, Guarda et al., 2007). Elzakkers et al. (2014) in their review of compulsory treatment conclude that, in the short term, there was no difference between voluntary and involuntarily treated patients. Also, at discharge treatment outcomes appear to be equivalent between those civilly committed and those treated on a voluntary basis. Clearly, there is no consensus on how civil commitment affects the therapeutic endeavor.

A study by Tan et al. (2010) may offer some insight based on the attitudes of individuals with anorexia nervosa and compulsory treatment. In their study, overall participants viewed civil commitment in general as supportive and helpful especially when the individual has diminished ability to understand and make decisions. When it came to saving a life, this group of individuals diagnosed with anorexia nervosa all agreed that overriding autonomy was imperative. In addition, many participants stated that, in retrospect, civil commitment had been warranted and accepted. Participants indicated that anorexia nervosa was part of their identity. Due to the illness and fear of loss of control, their personal values were changed and they experienced difficulties in judgment and decisions to accept treatment. These factors led to the need for more pressure to engage in effective treatment. These individuals also reported a positive perception of civil commitment when treatment decisions were transparent in the context of a good therapeutic relationship (Tan et al., 2010, Tan et al., 2003).

Tan, Stewart, and Hope (2009) point out that for those under civil commitment, it was the relationship and attitude of their health care professionals rather than freedom of choice that was of value during their treatment. During treatment, decisions based on mutual trust and confidence were more important than theoretical orientation or clinical practice. Some participants expressed that strong authority, pressure, and/or limits established by professionals indicated support and caring. These limitations also alleviated the need to make hard decisions on their own. The ultimate aspect for some participants was the development of trust with their treating professionals. When this occurred it helped the participant to reduce their defensiveness and misgivings about treatment and engage in the work of change (Tan et al., 2009). Resentment toward professionals was more likely to occur when a participant experienced being dismissed, belittled, or stripped of their individuality due to overly restrictive protocols.

From the perspective of the individual under civil commitment the outcome of that act seems a mixed bag. Loss of autonomy and disempowerment create more resistance to engagement in treatment, while development of a strong, trusting relationship with supportive flexible treatment protocols help them to feel more actively involved in their care.

A striking result was that what mattered most to participants was not whether they were compelled to have treatment but the nature of their relationships with parents and mental health professionals. Indeed, within a trusting relationship compulsion may be experienced as care (Tan et al., 2010, Tan et al., 2003).

Involvement of Parents and Significant Others

Data indicate that there is a significant impact on caregiver mental health, with the most disruption occurring between family and patient, especially among mothers and partners of the patient (Parks, Anastasiadou, Sánchez, Graell, & Sepulveda, 2017). Equally impaired is a poor quality of life for the caregiver and the increasing tension within the family due to assisting the patient to focus on change or treatment (Martín et al., 2011). The literature indicates that caregivers of individuals with eating disorders have substantial rates of anxiety and depression that seems to be sustained over at least one year (Orive et al., 2013). Also, the longer the duration of illness the more intense is the experience of distress (Martín et al., 2011, Parks et al., 2017). There does seem to be a reduction in caregiver distress when the caregiver spends less time with the afflicted individual (Martín et al., 2011, Parks et al., 2017). This might lend support for the need for temporarily removing the afflicted individual from the caregiver, which would most likely mean civil commitment.

In most cases involving eating disorders, by the time involuntary hospitalization and treatment is under consideration the patient will have been deemed incompetent and lacking decisional capacity. However, at some point, even the most profoundly caring family or significant other may find themselves inclined to violate an individuals' autonomy when the extent of their illness makes it impossible to maintain health. The consequence of those behaviors directs the family toward coercion. The perception of coercion in civil commitment is complex and not necessarily related to the degree of restriction of freedom. In thinking about and invoking compulsory treatment, we want to do what is right and good or at least what will be best for the greatest number (patient, family, significant others) (Kenney, 2012, Tansey, 2011).

Compulsory treatment can be viewed as being in the best interest of the patient but also for family and/or significant others. Orive et al. (2013) found that the majority of family caregivers experience a burden of caregiving in direct proportion to the perception of the patient's symptoms. The more intense the symptoms, the more distress experienced by the family. This distress effects the quality of life of caregiver and patient, leading to greater hostility and potentially a poor outcome (Parks et al., 2017). Invoking civil commitment could create emotional distance between the family and the patient's illness. Also, civil commitment and involuntary treatment offer an opportunity to help relatives understand the patient's problematic behaviors as symptoms of illness rather than misbehavior (Orive et al., 2013). When to use civil commitment becomes a serious decision often creating anguish for family and health care professionals. By the same token, the decision to use civil commitment and involuntary treatment reduces distress for the family or significant other and eliminates the sense of being helpless regarding the health of their loved one (Bowers, 2014).

The use of civil commitment by or for the family needs to professionally driven. This will work to reduce the potential for resentment and destruction of the relationship with or toward parents and possibly enhance communication between caregiver and affected individual (Tan et al., 2010). Goldner (1989) also identifies involvement of the family when considering civil commitment. The use of civil commitment can save distraught caregivers and help the family work toward a rational treatment plan. In addition, he perceives that civil commitment could reduce the negative influence asserted by the family during the time leading up to the decision regarding civil commitment (Goldner, 1989).

In considering the compassionate use of civil commitment, there needs to be a balanced, ethically principled approach that respects the dignity or autonomy of the affected person while working to prevent deterioration of the person's and caregiver's health. Respect for personal dignity does not rely on autonomy (allowing patients to make their own decisions) alone, but is also supported by the principles of beneficence (providing care that will benefit the patient), nonmaleficence (do no harm), and paternalism (interfering with a person's freedom for his or her own good; Kenney, 2012, Tansey, 2011). These principles can provide a compassionate stance for the patient and caregiver. Beneficence and paternalism can be seen as overruling autonomy (Kenney, 2012, Tansey, 2011), thereby establishing an opportunity for the individual with an eating disorder to create both short-term and long-term change. Without this chance the individual is likely to have continued interference with one's life goals and perhaps death. Additionally, making emotional room for caregivers increases the likelihood for a more positive short-term outcome (Parks et al., 2017). As noted earlier, people with AN appear to agree with the necessity of compulsory treatment in order to save life and this often extends anecdotally to the use of civil commitment by hospitalized patients (Watson, Bowers, & Andersen, 2000, Guarda et al., 2007). Compassionate use of civil commitment can also play an important role in treatment of eating disorders, strengthening the therapeutic bond (Tan et al., 2003, Watson et al., 2000).

References

Andersen, A.E. (2008). Ethical conflicts in the care of anorexia nervosa patients. *Eating Disorders Review*, 19, 1–4.

Andersen, A.E., Bowers, W., & Evans, K. (1997). Inpatient treatment of anorexia nervosa. *Handbook of Treatment for Eating Disorders*, 2, 327–353.

Bowers, W.A. (2014). Civil commitment in the treatment of eating disorders and substance abuse: Empirical status and ethical considerations. In T. Brewerton & A. Baker Dennis (Eds.) *Eating disorders, addictions and substance use disorders* (pp. 649–664). Berlin: Springer.

Caplan, A.L. (2006). Ethical issues surrounding forced, mandated, or coerced treatment. *Journal of Substance Abuse Treatment*, 31(2), 117–120.

Carney, T. (2014). The incredible complexity of being? Degrees of influence, coercion, and control of the "autonomy" of severe and enduring anorexia nervosa patients. *Journal of Bioethical Inquiry*, 11(1), 41–42.

Dresser, R. (1984a). Feeding the hunger artists: Legal issues in treating anorexia nervosa. *Wisconsin Law Review*, 297.

Dresser, R. (1984b). Legal and policy considerations in treatment of anorexia nervosa patients. *International Journal of Eating Disorders*, 3(4), 43–51.

Elzakkers, I.F., Danner, U.N., Hoek, H.W., Schmidt, U., & Elburg, A.A. (2014). Compulsory treatment in anorexia nervosa: A review. *International Journal of Eating Disorders*, 47(8), 845–852.

Fairburn, C.G. (2008). *Cognitive behavior therapy and eating disorder.* New York: Guilford Press.

Goldner, E. (1989). Treatment refusal in anorexia nervosa. *International Journal of Eating Disorders*, 8(3), 297–306.

Goldner, E.M., Birmingham, C.L., & Smye, V. (1997). Addressing treatment refusal in anorexia nervosa: Clinical, ethical, and legal considerations. In D.M. Garner & P.E. Garfinkel (Eds.), *Handbook of treatment for eating disorders*, 2, 450–461. New York: Guilford Press.

Guarda, A., Pinto, A., Coughlin, J., Hussain, S., Haug, N., & Heinberg, L. (2007). Perceived coercion and change in perceived need for admission in patients hospitalized for eating disorders. *American Journal of Psychiatry*, 164, 108–114.

Kenney, D.W. (2012). Making Gandhi Ji eat: Dare we? Workshop presented at the 4th Annual Eating Recovery Center Foundation Eating Disorders Conference, Denver, CO.

Martín, J., Padierna, A., Aguirre, U., Quintana, J.M., Las Hayas, C., & Muñoz, P. (2011). Quality of life among caregivers of patients with eating disorders. *Quality of Life Research*, 20(9), 1359–1369.

Mehler, P.S., & Andersen, A.E. (2017). *Eating disorders: A guide to medical care and complications* (3rd ed.). Baltimore, MD: Johns Hopkins Press.

Orive, M., Padierna, A., Martin, J., Aguirre, U., González, N., Muñoz, P., & Quintana, J.M. (2013). Anxiety and depression among caregivers of patients with eating disorders and their change over 1 year. *Social Psychiatry and Psychiatric Epidemiology*, 48(9), 1503–1512.

Parks, M., Anastasiadou, D., Sánchez, J.C., Graell, M., & Sepulveda, A.R. (2017). Experience of caregiving and coping strategies in caregivers of adolescents with an eating disorder: A comparative study. *Psychiatry Research*, 260, 241–247.

Russell, G.F. (2001). Involuntary treatment in anorexia nervosa. *Psychiatric Clinics of North America*, 24(2), 337–349.

Sheehan, K.A. (2009). Compulsory treatment in psychiatry. *Current Opinion in Psychiatry*, 22, 582–586.

Sheehan, K.A., & Burns, T. (2011). Perceived coercion and the therapeutic relationship: a neglected association? *Psychiatric Services*, 62(5), 471–476.

Silber, T.J. (2011). Treatment of anorexia nervosa against the patient's will: Ethical considerations. *Adolescent Medicine-State of the Art Reviews*, 22(2), 283.

Strober, M. (2006). Managing the chronic, treatment resistant patient with anorexia nervosa. *International Journal of Eating Disorders*, 36, 245–255.

Tan, J., & Richards, L. (2015). Legal and ethical issues in the treatment of really sick patients with anorexia nervosa. In *Critical care for anorexia nervosa* (pp. 113–150). Berlin: Springer International.

Tan, J.O., Hope, T., Stewart, A., & Fitzpatrick, R. (2003). Control and compulsory treatment in anorexia nervosa: The views of patients and parents. *International Journal of Law and Psychiatry*, 26(6), 627–645.

Tan, J.O., Stewart, A., Fitzpatrick, R., & Hope, T. (2010). Attitudes of patients with anorexia nervosa to compulsory treatment and coercion. *International Journal of Law and Psychiatry*, 33(1), 13–19.

Tan, J.O., Stewart, A., & Hope, T. (2009). Decision-making as a broader concept. *Philosophy, Psychiatry, & Psychology*, 16(4), 345–349.

Tansey, J. (2011). Ethical analysis: Civil commitment. Workshop presented at the 45th Association of Behavioral and Cognitive Therapy, Toronto, CA.

Watson, T.L., Bowers, W.A., & Andersen, A.E. (2000). Involuntary treatment of eating disorders. *American Journal of Psychiatry*, 157, 1806–1810.

Werth, J.L., Jr., Wright, K.S., Archambault, R.J., & Bardash, R.J. (2003). When does the "duty to protect" apply with a client who has anorexia nervosa? *Counseling Psychologist*, 31(4), 427–450.

Yager, J., Carney, T., & Touyz, S. (2016). Is involuntary (compulsory) treatment ever justified in patients with SE-AN: An international perspective. In S. Touyz, D. LeGrange, H. Lacey, & P. Hay (Eds.), *Managing severe and enduring anorexia nervosa: A clinician's guide* (pp. 185–201). Abingdon: Routledge.

7

Summary and Recommendations

Eating disorders have been described in the medical literature for hundreds of years. From the accounts of anorexia nervosa by Morton (Kaufman & Heiman, 1964) or the more concise descriptions by Gull and Lesaque in the 1880s (Kaufman & Herman, 1964) and Russell's (Russell, 1979) description of bulimia nervosa, we have been working to better understand and treat these complex and persistent disorders (Touyz & Hay, 2015). Without effective intervention these disorders lead to debilitating and possibly chronic medical complications (Westmoreland & Mehler, 2016), as well as severe and enduring psychological impediments (Touyz & Hay, 2015). Indeed, eating disorders disrupt family and social relationships and impede educational, financial, and employment goals (American Psychiatric Association, 2006). To that end, it is extremely important to consider all treatment possibilities when intervening with individuals with an eating disorder.

Eventually, some individuals find themselves in the grip of an illness that they can no longer stop or control. With help, many do regain control. But for a minority, the syndrome becomes enduring, with complete life disruption and potentially death (Touyz, LeGrange, Lacey, & Hay, 2015). At more advanced stages of the illness, fear of treatment and anxiety over loss of one's identity create an environment that undermines effective decision making. Additionally, overvalued ideas about weight and shape undercut capacity to make value-based decisions leading to treatment refusal and endangering life. Under such conditions, with proper therapeutic safeguards to preserve trust in the therapeutic alliance, it may be ethically appropriate to override decisions to refuse lifesaving treatment, even though individuals appear competent (Charland, 2013).

Of primary concern in civil commitment is the principle of autonomy. A time-honored idea in medicine, autonomy infers that individuals have control over their body and medical decision making. This central concept implies patient self-determination in medicine. However, in psychiatric disorders, when autonomy is compromised by a debilitating illness there is a need to override autonomy. In cases where life is threatened, the clinician's obligation to consider justified paternalism is considered acting in the patient's best interests. So while the individual's right to self-determination is acknowledged, a duty to protect requires a clinician to proceed with treatment even if this is against the patient's wishes (Andersen, 2008, Watson, Bowers, & Andersen 2000, Goldner, 1989). A supporting argument is that respect for self-determination sometimes requires mandatory treatment as a way to create or enable autonomy (Kenney, 2012, Tansey, 2011, Caplan, 2006).

The most paternalistic approach to helping an individual with an eating disorder is civil commitment. While it appears unethical to override an individual's right to choose the course of their care, it is in fact a most compassionate and truly beneficent approach. Andersen (2008) states that true beneficence is the heart of patient care. When overriding an individual's right to choose, ethical interventions arise from a comprehensive knowledge of an eating disorder and are based on experience and empirical evidence of what works. Paternalism can be diminished by the clinician's therapeutic skills and expression of empathy and acceptance, which validates the individual's struggles. Beneficence can provoke curiosity within the individual about the outcome of a healthy life. Additionally, a warm, nonjudgmental stance combined with unconditional positive regard establishes a challenge to the perceived benefits of the illness.

In the context of overriding an individual's right to choose another approach to ethical treatment is a full unambiguous disclosure of a professional's personal values. In addition, the health care provider must make transparent their rationale and steps involved in their decision making (Goldner, 1989). As such, civil commitment and involuntary treatment must be reasoned, ethical, and subject to rigorous standards. Kenney (2012) suggests contemplating the following questions when considering civil commitment:

1 Is this an end-of-life situation?
2 How will the patient benefit from treatment and will others benefit (i.e., family, providers, the community)?
3 How realistic are the treatment goals?
4 What criteria constitute success or failure?
5 What is the time frame for imposing the treatment?
6 What financial concerns exist for the patient or family?
7 What is our standard of care?
8 What does the literature suggest about the efficacy of involuntary treatment?

As can be seen, decisions to override an individual's autonomy must be based on a coherent discussion among professionals, family, and the distressed individual. Additional ethical principles or questions include: What makes civil commitment morally permissible, or morally repugnant? Is there a consensus for this decision? How is it morally permissible to force a person with a life-threatening mental disorder into treatment? Is the individual able to make competent decisions? (Kenney, 2012).

Understanding if the individual with an eating disorder can make competent decisions is often hard, as these individuals operate very well in day-to-day tasks (Carney, 2009). Seemingly, problems with decision making are narrow and focused on concerns regarding weight, adequate nutrition, and physical health. Rarely does the issue of competence focus on the individual's ambivalence regarding treatment. Introducing the concept of civil commitment can be seen as a method to reduce ambivalence about treatment, assist in changing false beliefs about weight, shape, and health, while restoring the person's autonomy to make appropriate health care decisions (Caplan, 2006, Kenney, 2012). If there is a decision to compel another person into treatment, this course of action must proceed with personal humility, cultural humility, professional humility, and awe of the dignity of the human person (Kenney, 2012).

Overriding autonomy that leads to civil commitment and compulsory treatment is usually initiated on the basis of dangerousness criterion or the need for treatment criterion indicating more severe status (Clausen & Jones, 2014). Ethical treatment of eating disorders must include civil commitment when there is a danger to physical and psychological life. When it is important to save a life, reduce the disruptive influence on family, and assist in creating a more valued life, overriding autonomy is ethically acceptable intervention (Kenney, 2012, Tansey, 2011). Overriding autonomy takes on many forms, including persuasion and coercion by way of legal methods.

The clinician must be aware of both the ethical and legal ramifications for civil commitment. Cooper (1976) advised clinicians to understand that the courts require the nature and duration of the commitment to bear some reasonable relation to the purposes for which the individual was committed. A better understanding of the determining factors and effect of involuntary treatment may necessitate difficult decisions for the clinician. Improved understanding of the determining factors regarding civil commitment help develop well-defined guidelines when deciding on involuntary treatment including consideration of the least restrictive environment for care (Clausen & Jones, 2014).

Positives of Civil Commitment

Although contested in the literature (Draper, 2000), there are positive aspects to civil commitment. Primary is intervention in a life-threatening illness. Civil commitment prevents life from being jeopardized (Tan, Hope, Stewart, & Fitzpatrick, 2003). Civil commitment also allows for medical stabilization which affects preservation of life and restoration of physical complications (Westmoreland & Mehler, 2016). Along the same line, civil commitment reduces the possibility of continued psychological harm. Civil commitment and involuntary treatment promote health and safety. Restoring the individual to normal physical status increases the prospect of challenging the overvalued beliefs surrounding the disorder (Westmoreland & Mehler, 2016). Overriding autonomy and creating an environment for treatment can also strengthen therapeutic alliance. Individuals have stated that they found involuntary treatment of great importance to a positive outcome (Guarda et al., 2007, Watson et al., 2000). In the same manner, patients identified civil commitment as a way of validating their need for treatment even when they experienced civil commitment as coercive (Tan, Stewart, Fitzpatrick, & Hope, 2010, Carney, 2009).

Therapeutic interventions emphasizing hope that recovery is possible can have some effect on low self-esteem and ineffectiveness, which predict poorer outcomes (Dawson, Rhodes, & Touyz,

2014). Civil commitment offers individuals opportunities to engage in treatment that will focus on a better quality of life and reduction in the debilitating aspects of an eating disorder (Touyz, Le Grange, Lacey, & Hay, 2016). Hope is continuously recognized as a key component in recovery from mental illness. It is deemed to be both activate the recuperation process and maintain movement toward recovery. An emphasis on internalizing improved quality of life and the value of change can create autonomy, thereby helping the individual shift away from eating disorder behavior. Personal awareness and support from others are factors implicated in the recovery process and both are important considerations for treatment. Overriding autonomy establishes opportunities to increase internal locus of control, which is important for the development of motivation to change. Patients with an eating disorder as well as clinicians must maintain the belief that recovery from an eating disorder is possible and civil commitment creates an environment that can reintroduce autonomy (Dawson et al., 2014). Patients' and clinicians' beliefs and attitudes about prognosis will have important implications for outcomes (Dawson et al., 2014).

Negatives of Civil Commitment

Use of civil commitment is passionately debated and negative features have been suggested (Draper, 2000, Ryan & Callaghan, 2014). A primary argument is that civil commitment violates a patient's right to decide (autonomy). Also, it has been contended that use of civil commitment and involuntary treatment does not actually treat the disorder. Successful treatment requires patient cooperation which is removed with civil commitment. One of the most intense claims is that civil commitment may create irreparable damage to the therapeutic relationship (Draper, 1998, Draper, 2000). With psychotherapy as the primary intervention in the treatment of eating disorders, civil commitment interferes with continued improvement for the patient. Along with a rift in the therapeutic relationship, involuntary treatment could reduce future desire for the patient to remain in treatment. A final contention is that civil commitment does not assure improvement in the disorder past medical stabilization, leaving few if no long-term positive outcomes (Goldner, McKenzie, & Kline 1991).

Grisso and Appelbaum (1995) advocate the ethical importance of decisional capacity. There must be an assessment of a patient's ability to communicate a choice and the ability to understand information relevant to making treatment decisions in regard to overriding autonomy. Along with the ability to communicate and understand decision making, the patient must have the ability to appreciate the significance of the information presented and how to apply it to one's own situation (e.g., insight). Also, the patient must have the ability to reason with relevant information and to participate in logical reasoning and weighing options regarding care and self-determination of their needs. These concepts must be employed when considering civil commitment or overriding autonomy.

Another ethical discussion is regarding informed consent. Does an individual with an eating disorder who refuses treatment and has autonomy overridden engage in treatment via informed consent? Beauchamp and Childress (2001) suggest a standard for informed consent. This would include disclosure of all information by the health care worker and the patients understanding of all information regarding care. To avoid coercion and minimize bias, the patient must voluntarily accept this information and be stable to authorize and make choices. Additionally, informed consent must be questioned when a patient refuses treatment, particularly in the face of a likely adverse outcome. In essence involuntary treatment does not meet their idea of informed consent, making it hard to justify. Civil commitment would be a procedure that did not qualify as informed consent.

Clinicians must be alert to the impact of their own feelings and biases on their actions. They must guard against stigmatization or minimization especially when patients are viewed as difficult to treat or personally distressing to manage. Clinicians must be knowledgeable, responsive, and flexible in their understanding of the impact of eating disorders on decisions to accept or refuse treatment. They must be aware of the needs and preferences of their patient regarding decision making for themselves or with others. Clinicians must be compassionate and empathetic when overriding autonomy and be alert to reducing the influence of coercion when treatment becomes difficult (Tan & Richards, 2015).

Persuasion or Coercion

In a treatment setting, persuasion ranges from mild interventions such as requests or reasoning to stronger forms like bargaining, gentle prodding, enticement, selective information, or manipulation. Persuasion as an aspect of therapy can be adopted to obtain treatment compliance. It can be utilized during communication between health care provider and patient when detailing options and/or strategies related to treatment goals. Generally, persuasion is seen as a method to help a patient focus on the best decisions regarding their care.

Coercion in a clinical setting is also made up of many variables, and like persuasion it relies on the forms of communication between clinician and patient. However, coercion reflects the potential of inequality of power based on the patient's knowledge of their options when it comes to taking charge of their care or presenting their wishes that are contrary to the health care provider, the family, or the state. When the patient's goals create a life-threatening situation, coercion can be seen as a legitimate model to deliver care. However, the use of coercion dramatically closes down the size of the remaining decisional "space" within which a person still retains the power of choice. Coercion either limits choice or creates the illusion of choice and limits or overrides an individual's autonomy to make medical decisions. Herein lies the ethical dilemma in the treatment of individuals with eating disorders.

Coercive treatment can be ethically justified in a very limited number of cases as a last resort and under strict conditions. Decisions about involuntary commitment should be based on a capacity criterion, not on an illness or dangerousness criterion. Coercive treatment can be justified as being in the interest of the patient according to his or her presumed values and preferences, not as being in the interest of others. If dangerous behaviors are expected to give rise to loss of freedom and social exclusion, providing treatment that is expected to prevent these outcomes and improve the illness is in the patient's interest. The mental illness criterion should be replaced by a capacity criterion, allowing short-term detention for purposes of assessment in cases of uncertainty (Steinert, 2016). Involuntary detention or imposed treatment is not ordinary treatment; it may provide the opportunity to preserve life, but it can have anti-therapeutic effects which also need to be considered (Carney, Tait, & Touyz, 2007).

Ethical Considerations

Coercion via civil commitment and involuntary treatment demands understanding of the ethical considerations that are foundation of all clinical treatment. As such, ethical aspects of coercion fall into the same realms as any other medical treatment. Primary and the most debated ethical concerns are: autonomy (freedom of choice;

allowing patients to make their own decisions), paternalism (interfering with a person's freedom for his or her own good), nonmaleficence ("do no harm"), beneficence (providing care that will benefit the patient), and justice (Striving for fairness).

When coercion is introduced into treatment, it is important to understand how interventions move toward ethical excellence regarding therapy goals and outcome. Good clinical and ethical practice must include respecting the patient's autonomy and use the least restrictive interventions. Broadly, ethical excellence in treatment of eating disorders requires intervention strategies that are both effective and meaningful. A helpful treatment perspective is that patients are inherently part of the treatment solution. Therefore, ethical treatment strives to make the treatment and change process collaborative. Clinicians may create interventions in the name of good practice and the best interest of the patient, but the most competent professional risks losing sight of the individual. We cannot be effective in our care if we do not understand the patient's perspective.

Alleviation of coercion can be accomplished by an "ethics of caring" approach (Andersen, 2008). This approach proposes that effective patient care is embedded in healing relationships. The quality of the relationship between patients and professionals becomes the basis for sound decision making in the treatment of eating disorders. With a good relationship, patients who do not consider having a choice do not necessarily resent their experiences nor perceive them as coercive; instead they view the strong influence, pressure, supervision, or restrictions imposed by professionals as helpful, caring, and supportive (Watson et al., 2000, Guarda, 2008). Most patients eventually see that the treatment against their wishes is justified and there is very little resentment of sense of coercion (Watson et al., 2000, Guarda, 2008). However, resentment is expressed when patients sense that their wishes and who they are has been dismissed or they were punitively treated. Alternatively, other patients can resent supervision and restriction imposed on them and view the restrictions as having been unhelpful in their process of recovery (Tan et al., 2010).

A key reason patients reported resentment was the rigidity of treatment regimens that ignored their wishes, disregarded personal choice, and deprived them of their individuality. Patients indicated that poor relationships with professionals were the result of punitive, dismissive, or disrespectful behavior and failure of the professional to listen carefully and respectfully to their feelings and wishes. Perceived indifference of professionals was more disruptive than restriction of choice. Of central importance to patients was not whether the treatment was seen as in their best interest or the best course of action, but whether the patients were able to trust the professionals enough to overcome their own ambivalence and reservations (Tan, et al., 2003).

Coercion can and does occur in the treatment of individuals with an eating disorder. As such, ethical issues must not be at the margin of treatment. Concern and awareness of ethics must be incorporated into the all aspects of care to reduce the impact of coercion. Reduction in the impact of coercion can be fostered by the following these ethical standards:

1 Respect autonomy (when possible encourage joint decision making)

2 Use paternalism sparingly (when possible limit interference in personal freedom)

3 Nonmaleficence

4 Beneficence (use interventions that have been shown to be effective)

5 Stay collaborative in treatment and goals

6 Validate the individual's fears, beliefs, and concerns

7 Utilize unconditional positive regard

8 Accept and validate the patient is doing the best they can

9 Remain transparent with your professional and personal values about treatment

10 Share your rationale about how you make decisions.

(Kenney, 2012, Tansey, 2011)

Keeping these principles in mind can reduce the distress of civil commitment and involuntary treatment. Additionally, perceived coercion is not a constant and fluctuates over the course of treatment. Patients have also identified the nature of their treatment relationship as a cushion to coercion. A relationship that was perceived as nonjudgmental and validated their struggle was seen as more important than whether they were compelled or coerced to have treatment. Within a trusting relationship coercion may be experienced as care (Andersen, 2007).

Patient Viewpoint

Patients want to be seen as unique individuals with room for their personal situations as part of their recovery. Patients are also critical of what seems to be an overemphasis on target weights. Weight is usually seen as the least important part of successful treatment. Patients come into conflict when clinicians see weight restoration as a sign of recovery and miss that the thoughts or beliefs about weight, shape, size, appearance, and food must be shifted to create enduring change. Additionally, patients experience treatment as being rushed when their voice is not acknowledged or heard. Coercion in creating unilateral goals undermines the likelihood of acceptance. Additionally, lack of transparency in treatment goals and refusal to listen block progress. Clinicians must strive to create a collaborative approach to treatment by working to meet where they are at and meet the individual's needs. When this is accomplished, patients report in hindsight that they were grateful for their care (Watson et al., 2000, Guarda et al., 2007).

Alternatives to Civil Commitment

Psychiatric Advanced Directives

Psychiatric advanced directives (PAD) are one potential mechanism available to individuals with anorexia nervosa to help minimize many of the ambiguities commonly associated with mental health crises. PADs are legal documents that allow competent individuals, through advance instructions, and or designation of a health care agent, to declare preferences for future mental health treatment when they may not be capable of doing so as the result of a psychiatric crisis. Having a PAD may be a way to avoid or reduce involuntary treatment in the hospital. PADs are potentially helpful for several reasons. First, they can enable consumers to assume control over treatment decisions. Second, they can be used to enhance communications about treatment preferences between patients, families, and health care providers. Third, a PAD may expedite appropriate and timely treatment interventions before situations deteriorate to emergency status. Fourth, they may lead to reductions in adversarial court proceedings over involuntary psychiatric treatment. Developing a PAD may improve autonomy, decrease the need for coercive interventions, and enrich clinical outcomes through clarity in provision of preferred services during a crises. Enhanced engagement in the treatment process, improved self-efficacy, and personal empowerment could result from an individual developing a PAD.

Severe and Enduring Eating Disorders

The American Psychiatric Association (APA, 2006) treatment guidelines suggests efforts to understand the unique plight of patients with a severe and enduring form of an eating disorder (SEED). Utilization of a more supportive model of treatment with less emphasis on behavioral change and weight gain is recommended. Treatment emphasis is on maximizing medical stability, quality of life, and social relationships. Psychotherapeutic procedures are core interventions designed to engage and motivate the patient. This model emphasizes the development of compassionate care relying on the therapeutic alliance to foster better nutritional rehabilitation while emphasizing fewer relapses and smaller weight restoration (Touyz & Hay, 2015, Strober, 2006, Touyz et al., 2016).

Therapeutic interventions must establish reasonable goals that are acceptable to the patient, family, and health care team. Also, conditions under which family members would be contacted and circumstances leading to an imposition of civil commitment must be clearly understood by all members of the team, the patient, and the family. Clear guidelines regarding symptom status and case management services may also enhance long-term care. However, the severity of some patients' disorders, their need for autonomy, or difficulty collaborating may make long-term care impossible. When the patient who is not focused on active symptom change is hospitalized, hospital-based teams must individualize treatment protocols. This is complicated, given many hospital-based programs are focused on weight restoration and psychotherapy. In these cases the focus of care is on medical stability and maintenance goals. With proper supervision, most medical complications can be managed in an inpatient eating disorder treatment setting.

Patients with SEED may require short-term hospitalizations on medical units. Ideally, medical stabilization units would have available staff who are well trained in the needs of individuals with a chronic eating disorder. The focus on care remains on medical stability rather than expectations for full recovery. If medical units are used, once medical stabilization is reached, these patients should be transferred to an eating disorder unit. In this type of environment psychiatric and nutritional interventions can be implemented, as well as step-down to outpatient care.

Yager, Carney, and Touyz (2016) suggest when a patient's medical or psychological status deteriorates there is a role for overriding consent and autonomy. If hospitalization occurs the treatment milieu must encourage patients to become effectively involved in their treatment and enable them to make informed choices in the least restrictive environment (Touyz and Carney, 2010). This type of intervention is designed to protect a patient's rights and well-being (Touyz & Hay, 2015, Touyz & Strober, 2016). Clinicians must be mindful that this approach (which can include involuntary treatment) needs to be collaborative and health care teams must understand the personal directives of the patient. Thiels (2008) has concluded that enforced hospitalization of a patient with severe and enduring eating disorder is not only necessary but ethically responsible.

Care of individuals with a severe and enduring eating disorder have a major emphasis on the patient's quality of life (Bamford et al., 2015). Treatment should not shift entirely away from weight and symptom change onto improved quality of life. Additionally, clinicians must communicate to patients that improvements in quality of life may be unlikely without change in weight, and progress in psychological, and behavioral eating disorder symptoms. Improvement in BMI and reduction of eating disorder symptoms remains important but secondary to quality of life. Interventions that balance between improved symptoms and enhanced quality of life may be more effective in achieving improvements in both domains (Bamford et al., 2015).

Ethics and Civil Commitment

Given the disruption of one's personal life and the potential life-threatening aspects of an eating disorder, clinicians, families, and patients must understand the unforgiving nature of this illness. To balance the wishes of the patient and treatment team, it is ethically important to adjust the usual treatment model (Yager, 2007, Touyz et al., 2015, Strober, 2006), especially with those suffering from a severe and enduring form of the illness. These adjustments will include civil commitment, harm reduction, and perhaps palliative care (Westmoreland & Mehler, 2016). When civil commitment is considered, rarely is there a viable advanced directive based on the patient's clear decisional capacity. The decision then to treat involuntarily must be subjected to a thorough ethical examination. What process can we depend upon before deciding on involuntary hospitalization and treatment? Also, what questions need to be embraced to make an ethically informed decision when overriding autonomy?

The primary question in civil commitment is, is this an end-of-life situation? When one's life is in jeopardy, states allow for *parens patriae* to be invoked. Dangerousness to oneself or others will be sufficient to override autonomy (Carney, 2009). If a patient's clinical condition meets common legal criteria for involuntary admission to hospital and treatment, there is no reason individuals with an eating disorder should be excluded from consideration for lifesaving treatment (Andersen, 2007, Tan & Richards, 2015, Yager et al., 2016). Are loved ones, providers, and other caregivers to be included in this decision? This is often the case, as both health care providers and family members typically establish the momentum for civil commitment. Will the patient benefit from treatment? While this can be debated based on the outcome of treatment, most patients gain short-term benefits from civil commitment and involuntary treatment (Elzakkers, Danner, Hoek, Schmidt, & Elburg, 2014, Watson et al., 2000, Guarda et al., 2007). It is the longer-term outcomes that are often questioned (Ramsay, Ward, Treasure, & Russell, 1999, Watson et al., 2000, Brunner, Parzer, & Resch, 2005, Thiel & Paul, 2007).

Other ethical questions to be addressed are, are the treatment goals realistic, and how will success be determined? This demands an understanding of the literature and the best empirically based treatment. What is the standard of care? Although there is little to address this, the APA guidelines for the treatment of eating and disorders and empirically based papers establish minimum criteria for treatment. What does the medical literature suggest about the efficacy of involuntary treatment? The existing literature suggests that in the short term there is a rationale for civil commitment and involuntary care. What time frame may be agreed upon for imposing the treatment? The time frame must be related to the goals of care but needs to accommodate treatment in the least restrictive environment. Do any of the participants have a conscientious objection to providing or withholding involuntary treatment? This would be an area where family or significant others must be part of the decision making process (Kenney, 2012, Tansey, 2011). These are the questions and tasks that must be considered when overriding autonomy.

Draper (2000) advocates a position that some suffering from anorexia nervosa are competent to refuse therapy. As such, the clinician must listen to the reasons given for their refusal. There is a need to see the difference between saving the life of a sufferer and curing them of their anorexia. The clinician must understand the burden that life with anorexia and therapy have become.

Involuntary treatment may be lifesaving, but it does not always change the underlying condition. In fact, Draper (2000) suggests it may make the disorder worse. Respecting a patient's autonomy in not simply about letting them make some decisions; it is about accepting that it is the patient who is responsible for the consequences of those decisions, not the person who seeks to intercede on their behalf. Carney (2009), on the other hand, feels it is hard to reject a role for law in the authorization of the use of coercion in some form. This is especially true in the case of emergency or lifesaving interventions for severe anorexia. Fedyszyn and Sullivan (2007) argue that ethical excellence in treatment of an eating disorder calls for intervention strategies that are both effective and meaningful. Ethical excellence focuses on empirically based treatment and interventions that follow the current best practice. This requires recognition for the psychological and physical complexity of an eating disorders that are only now being addressed by our clinical practice guidelines. Of great importance is the recognition of a spectrum of treatment needs for eating disorder patients. Included in this recognition is the appraisal of the effects of the illness, his/her readiness to change, and the duration of the illness. Also of importance is the recognition of our treatments and how well they serve the patient's needs and goals. They state that successful interventions must understand the benefits as well as the limitations of treatment to ethically implement care (Fedyszyn & Sullivan, 2007).

Kendall and Hugman (2014) focus on the ethics of treatment related to professional practice. Clinicians must be held accountable for their care and decisions through shared communication. They assert that team meetings are a necessary ethical forum where professionals demonstrate competence and expertise in the care and treatment of eating disorders. This view maintains that respect for autonomy should be applied along with social justice. This view honors the value of life with dignity. To achieve and support patient's values, treatment teams must hear and acknowledge patient perspectives. This mean that opportunities must be created for patient experience to be heard in team discussions. Additionally, treatment teams must be transparent. This transparency enables the patient to have some control within the treatment environment. Ethical care offers the patient information on how and why treatment decisions were made.

Although not specifically tied to ethical issues, Tan et al. (2003) advance Kendall and Hugman (2014) regarding transparency and awareness about the patient's struggles. A core issue for those diagnosed with anorexia nervosa is to be in control. This struggle in turn influences the patients' ability to accept treatment and has implications for the issue of compulsory treatment. Treatment teams must not lose sight of how impaired decision making may be due to this internal struggle. Also, clinicians must remain aware how the struggle affects the individual's understanding and reasoning. Treatment teams working from this ethical base hear and acknowledge a patient's struggle and its effects on patient decision making. Healing can be defined as a time when the patient's sense of self is no longer divided, which is often facilitated through therapy and close relationships (Jenkins & Ogden, 2012).

Emphasis on "Compassionate Compulsory Treatment"

For What Period of Time Should Someone Be Committed?

More severe presentations of eating disorder symptoms combined with complex comorbidities of Axis I and II disorders characterize the group that is most likely to need involuntary treatment. Civil commitment can be part of a comprehensive treatment plan. Blatant paternalism and disregard for autonomy are intended primarily to preserve life and health while overriding the intentions and fears of those struggling with the disorder. But what can be a more vexing question is how to implement the use of civil commitment in a longer-term perspective. Once the individual is deemed unable to make competent decisions and by virtue of those decisions they place their life in danger. As a result immediate intervention must occur. However, how long does the commitment need to be in place and what aspects of treatment must be accomplished to consider withdrawing the civil commitment? This is a more difficult question to answer.

The need to restore the individual to a minimum of health would include weight restoration to above a point at which the diagnosis can be made. Most programs and the APA suggest that the individual must attain a healthy normal weight. Although not clearly defined, this would be anywhere between a BMI of 18.5 and 25. This range can be problematic, as many who struggle with an eating disorder have a strong emotional focus on numbers and see a BMI above 19 as detrimental or outright scary. Given that these clinical features may in fact contribute to the maintenance of eating disorders, incorporating patient preferences into treatment selection among individuals with eating disorders may be especially problematic and complicate treatment outcome (Peterson, Becker, Treasure, Shafran, & Bryant-Waugh, 2016).

Also, there is no adequate definition of how long one must maintain a healthy normal weight to see the physical and psychological benefits of restoration. Limited data suggest that relapse or return to a more intense level of care (readmission to hospital from a partial hospital setting) is more likely if the individual is transitioned prior to restoring to at least 90% of health normal. This implies that a person must be maintained at least at this level to increase their odds of remaining on a positive recovery trajectory.

That being said, it would make sense that civil commitment be extended as least to this weight threshold. However, a reference point of 90% of healthy normal could be at odds with the dangerousness aspect of civil commitment. At what point does an individual move across the threshold of not being dangerous? When weight and medical criteria return to normal, it could be argued that the individual is out of danger. However, an equally compelling argument can be made for a psychological threshold to be attained, which would then have the concept of "grave disability" being more important than physical status. Observation of long-term outcome for the treatment of eating disorders could support this notion, which then maintains the civil commitment for a much longer time period. In essence, how long do you maintain someone on civil commitment status? This is a very hard question to answer for many reasons. Primary among them are that each state and perhaps each judge or magistrate interprets the dangerousness aspect of the law differently. Additionally, even though most states and provinces have laws that govern civil commitment that emphasize inpatient treatment, these primarily focus on dangerousness, and not all jurisdictions have laws that sustain that commitment to an outpatient basis (assisted outpatient treatment, or AOT). By mid-2016, 46 states and the District of Columbia had AOT laws on the books. But, within those states, AOT is still not the routine and universally available practice it ought to be (www. treatmentadvocacycenter.org).

The length of time a person can be maintained in civil commitment is determined by the law of each state, province, or country. As such a clinical must understand the limitations of civil commitment in their area. However, the little data that exist that might guide treatment suggest that maintaining a patient above a BMI of 19 for the year after discharge from an inpatient program enhances the chance of sustain improvement (Kaplan et al., 2009). Using these data, if it is possible, keeping an outpatient commitment for one year might be of value. However, it is also important to understand that maintaining a patient at such a BMI might be evidence that dangerousness is no longer a viable aspect to sustain the commitment. So this "double edged sword" of keeping someone in treatment via legal methods might diminish as your help the patient recover. Also, it is important to remember that treatment must be in the least restrictive environment so ethical care would question maintaining a commitment when there is no evidence to override autonomy.

Although the use of civil commitment is seen as an intervention of last resort perhaps in the treatment of eating disorders dangerousness as a primary reason must be questioned. Would our treatment be better served if it was not implemented at a point where the primary focus is to save a life or reverse the negative consequences of starvation? Perhaps it would be more important to focus on grave disability as a primary concept when considering civil commitment. If this were implemented perhaps we could prevent some of the irreversible aspect of a severe eating disorder. Also, treatment might be more effective if the individual who is under civil commitment and involuntary treatment had more of an opportunity to effectively use the therapy then one in a starved state. Additionally, a grave disability concept might lend treatment to less intense or restrictive treatment environments such as intensive outpatient care, partial hospital, or residential treatment.

Civil commitment is an important aspect of care of those individuals who are overwhelmed by an eating disorder. It is a hard clinical decision and must be addressed in an ethical manner which incorporates family desires, treatment goals, and prevention of physical and psychological maladies as well as input from the patient. While it is hard to override the wishes of our patients, at times this is the only viable option. It takes courage to help our patients return to health and a valued life, even when it means overriding their autonomy and power to make decisions.

References

American Psychiatric Association. (2006). Treatment of patients with eating disorders (3rd ed.). *American Journal of Psychiatry*, 163(7 Suppl), 4–54.

Andersen, A. (2007). Eating disorders and coercion. *American Journal of Psychiatry*, 164, 9–11.

Andersen, A.E. (2008). Ethical conflicts in the care of anorexia nervosa patients. *Eating Disorders Review*, 19, 1–4.

Bamford, B., Barras, C., Sly, R., Stiles-Shields, C., Touyz, S., Grange, D., . . . Lacey, H. (2015). Eating disorder symptoms and quality of life: Where should clinicians place their focus in severe and enduring anorexia nervosa? *International Journal of Eating Disorders*, 48(1), 133.

Beauchamp, T.L., & Childress, J.F. (2001). *Principles of biomedical ethics*. Oxford: Oxford University Press.

Brunner, R., Parzer, P., & Resch, F. (2005). Involuntary hospitalization of patients with anorexia nervosa: Clinical issues and empirical findings. *Fortschritte der Neurologie-Psychiatrie*, 73(1), 9–15.

Caplan, A.L. (2006). Ethical issues surrounding forced, mandated, or coerced treatment. *Journal of Substance Abuse Treatment*, 31(2), 117–120.

Carney, T. (2009). Anorexia: A role for law in therapy? *Psychiatry, Psychology and Law*, 16(1), 41–59.

Carney, T., Tait, D., & Touyz, S. (2007). Coercion is coercion? Reflections on trends in the use of compulsion in treating anorexia nervosa. *Australasian Psychiatry*, 15(5), 390–395.

Charland, L.C. (2013). Ethical and conceptual issues in eating disorders. *Current Opinion in Psychiatry*, 26(6), 562–565.

Clausen, L., & Jones, A. (2014). A systematic review of the frequency, duration, type and effect of involuntary treatment for people with anorexia nervosa, and an analysis of patient characteristics. *Journal of Eating Disorders*, 2(1), 29.

Cooper, G.G. (1976). Civil commitment of mentally ill; Right to treatment; Parens patriae power; Right to liberty; Donaldson v. O'Connor. *Akron Law Review*, 9(2), 9.

Dawson, L., Rhodes, P., & Touyz, S. (2014). "Doing the Impossible": The process of recovery from chronic anorexia nervosa. *Qualitative Health Research*, 24(4), 494–505.

Draper, H. (1998). Treating anorexics without consent: Some reservations. *Journal of Medical Ethics*, 24(1), 5.

Draper, H. (2000). Anorexia nervosa and respecting a refusal of life-prolonging therapy: A limited justification. *Bioethics*, 14(2), 120–133.

Elzakkers, I.F., Danner, U.N., Hoek, H.W., Schmidt, U., & Elburg, A.A. (2014). Compulsory treatment in anorexia nervosa: A review. *International Journal of Eating Disorders*, 47(8), 845–852.

Fedyszyn, I.E., & Sullivan, G.B. (2007). Ethical re-evaluation of contemporary treatments for anorexia nervosa: Is an aspirational stance possible in practice? *Australian Psychologist*, 42(3), 198–211.

Goldner, E. (1989). Treatment refusal in anorexia nervosa. *International Journal of Eating Disorders*, 8(3), 297–306.

Goldner, E.M., McKenzie, J.M., & Kline, S.A. (1991). The ethics of forced feeding in anorexia nervosa. *CMAJ: Canadian Medical Association Journal*, 144(10), 1205.

Grisso, T., & Appelbaum, P.S. (1995). Comparison of standards for assessing patients' capacities to make treatment decisions. *American Journal of Psychiatry*, 152(7), 1033.

Guarda, A., Pinto, A., Coughlin, J., Hussain, S., Haug, N., & Heinberg, L. (2007). Perceived coercion and change in perceived need for admission in patients hospitalized for eating disorders. *American Journal of Psychiatry*, 164, 108–114.

Guarda, A.S. (2008). Treatment of anorexia nervosa: Insights and obstacles. *Physiology & Behavior*, 94(1), 113–120.

Jenkins, J., & Ogden, J. (2012). Becoming "whole" again: A qualitative study of women's views of recovering from anorexia nervosa. *European Eating Disorders Review*, 20(1), 23–31.

Kaplan, A.S., Walsh, B.T., Olmsted, M., Attia, E., Carter, J.C., Devlin, M.J., . . . Parides, M. (2009). The slippery slope: Prediction of successful weight maintenance in anorexia nervosa. *Psychological Medicine*, 39, 1037–1045.

Kaufman, R.M., & Heiman, M.E. (1964). *Evolution of psychosomatic concepts*. New York: International Universities Press.

Kendall, S., & Hugman, R. (2014). Power/Knowledge and the ethics of involuntary treatment for anorexia nervosa in context: A social work contribution to the debate. *British Journal of Social Work*, 46(3), 686–702.

Kenney, D.W. (2012). Making Gandhi Ji eat: Dare we? Workshop presented at the 4th annual Eating Recovery Center Foundation Eating Disorders Conference, Denver, CO.

Peterson, C.B., Becker, C.B., Treasure, J., Shafran, R., & Bryant-Waugh, R. (2016). The three-legged stool of evidence-based practice in eating disorder treatment: Research, clinical, and patient perspectives. *BMC Medicine*, 14(1), 69.

Ramsay, R., Ward, A., Treasure, J., & Russell, G.F. (1999). Compulsory treatment in anorexia nervosa: Short-term benefits and long-term mortality. *British Journal of Psychiatry*, 175(2), 147–153.

Russell, G. (1979). Bulimia nervosa: An ominous variant of anorexia nervosa. *Psychological Medicine*, 9, 429–448.

Ryan, C.J., & Callaghan, S. (2014). Treatment refusal in anorexia nervosa: The hardest of cases. *Journal of Bioethical Inquiry*, 11(1), 43–45.

Steinert, T. (2016). Ethics of coercive treatment and misuse of psychiatry. *Psychiatric Services*, 68(3), 291–294.

Strober, M. (2006). Managing the chronic, treatment resistant patient with anorexia nervosa. *International Journal of Eating Disorders*, 36, 245–255.

Tan, J.O., Hope, T., Stewart, A., & Fitzpatrick, R. (2003). Control and compulsory treatment in anorexia nervosa: The views of patients and parents. *International Journal of Law and Psychiatry*, 26(6), 627–645.

Tan, J.O., Stewart, A., Fitzpatrick, R., & Hope, T. (2010). Attitudes of patients with anorexia nervosa to compulsory treatment and coercion. *International Journal of Law and Psychiatry*, 33(1), 13–19.

Tan, J., & Richards, L. (2015). Legal and ethical issues in the treatment of really sick patients with anorexia nervosa. In *Critical care for anorexia nervosa* (pp. 113–150). Berlin: Springer International.

Tansey, J. (2011). Ethical analysis: Civil commitment. Workshop presented at the 45th Association of Behavioral and Cognitive Therapy, Toronto, CA.

Thiel, A., & Paul, T. (2007). Compulsory treatment in anorexia nervosa. *Psychotherapie, Psychosomatik, Medizinische Psychologie, 57*(3–4), 128–135.

Thiels, C. (2008). Forced treatment of patients with anorexia. *Current Opinion in Psychiatry, 21*(5), 495–498.

Touyz, S.W., & Carney, T. (2010). Compulsory (involuntary) treatment for anorexia nervosa. In C.M. Grilo, & J.E. Mitchell (Eds.), *The treatment of eating disorders: A clinical handbook* (pp. 212–224). New York: Guilford Press.

Touyz, S., & Hay, P. (2015). Severe and enduring anorexia nervosa (SE-AN): In search of a new paradigm. *Journal of Eating Disorders, 3*(1), 26.

Touyz, S., Le Grange, D., Lacey, H., & Hay, P. (Eds.). (2016). *Managing severe and enduring anorexia nervosa: A clinician's guide.* Abingdon: Routledge.

Touyz, S., & Strober, M. (2016). Managing the patient with severe and enduring anorexia nervosa. In S. Touyz, D. LeGrange, H. Lacey, & P. Hay (Eds.), *Managing severe and enduring anorexia nervosa: A clinician's guide* (pp. 95–111). Abingdon: Routledge.

Watson, T.L., Bowers, W.A., & Andersen, A.E. (2000). Involuntary treatment of eating disorders. *American Journal of Psychiatry, 157,* 1806–1810.

Westmoreland, P., & Mehler, P.S. (2016). Caring for patients with severe and enduring eating disorders (SEED): Certification, harm reduction, palliative care, and the question of futility. *Journal of Psychiatric Practice, 22*(4), 313–320.

Yager, J. (2007). Management of patients with chronic, intractable eating disorders. *Clinical Manual of Eating Disorders,* 407–439.

Yager, J., Carney, T., & Touyz, S. (2016). Is involuntary (compulsory) treatment ever justified in patients with SE-AN: An international perspective. In S. Touyz, D. LeGrange, H. Lacey, & P. Hay (Eds.), *Managing severe and enduring anorexia nervosa: A clinician's guide* (pp. 185–201). Abingdon: Routledge.

Index

access to treatment 70–72
accountability for care, transfer of 42
ACTS (Assertive Community Treatment) 87
advanced directives: competence 79–84, 91, 93–94; legal recognition of 79, 81; *see also* psychiatric advanced directive
advanced psychiatric directives 32
alkalosis 7
American Psychiatric Association 40, 81, 124, 127, 130
anorexia nervosa: autonomy compromised by disorder 63, 65; civil commitment 45; coercion 45–47; cognitive dysfunction 9; demographics 1; described in literature 1–2; diagnosis 1; mortality rate 5, 8–9, 33–34; origin of term 2; patient attitudes toward compulsory treatment 103–104, 107; prevalence, onset, and course 4–5; psychiatric advanced directive 83; refusal of care 127, 129; severe and enduring anorexia nervosa (SE-AN) 11–13, 86–90; symptoms 1
AOT *see* assisted outpatient treatment
Assertive Community Treatment (ACTS) 87
assisted outpatient treatment (AOT) 23–24, 131
asylums 20–21
Australia, civil commitment in 26
autonomy 42, 124; client-centered approach to maintain 87; compassionate use of civil commitment and 100–105, 107; compromised by eating disorder 63,

65–67; Convention on the Rights of Persons with Disabilities (CRPD) and 29; ethical considerations 59–68, 70, 73, 119–121, 126–128; outpatient commitment 54; overriding by civil commitment 48–49, 51–52, 62, 64–66, 70, 73, 101–103, 112–119, 125–127, 130, 132; psychiatric advanced directive and 87–89, 91–94, 123; respect for 33, 63–64, 121, 128; restoration of 52, 62–63, 67, 114, 116; supportive decision making 32

Barrett's esophagus 7
behavioral contract, collaborative 86, 88
beneficence 33, 52, 60–64, 68, 70, 73, 100, 107, 112–113, 120–121
bingeing 3–4, 7, 53, 100–101
Binswanger, Ludwig 3
body image distortion 1, 3–5, 10
body mass index (BMI) 43, 125, 130–132
Boskind-Lodahl, Marlene 4
bulimarexia 4
bulimia nervosa: characteristic features of 3–4; descriptions in literature 3–4; mortality rate 8; prevalence, onset, and course 4–5; similarities to anorexia nervosa 3–4

Canada, civil commitment in 26–27
capacity 29–30, 34, 105; of adolescents 41; compromised by the eating disorders 102–103; ethical importance of 117; judicial determination of 82–83; psychiatric advanced directive and 82–85, 93–94

Index

caregivers: compassionate use of civil commitment 105–107; inclusion in decision 126–127; psychiatric advanced directives and 93
CBT (cognitive-behavioral therapy) 72, 90
chaotic eating 6, 9
civil commitment: alternatives to 123; anorexia nervosa patient attitudes toward 103–104, 107; autonomy overridden by 48–49, 51–52, 62, 64–66, 70, 73, 101–103, 112–119, 125–127, 130, 132; coercion 60, 105; compassionate use of 52, 99–107, 129–132; criticism of 48–49, 51, 59; damage to therapeutic relationship 116–117; eating disorders and 40–54; ethical considerations 59–73, 126–129; history of 19–36; individuals with eating disorders 33–34; influence on outpatient treatment 43; inhibiting the therapeutic relationship by 103; international 25–29; involvement of parents and significant others 105–107; modern 34–36; negatives of 116–118; outcome of 45–46, 51–52, 59–60, 103, 127; outpatient 52–54; patient view of 44–46; positives of 115–116; psychiatric advanced directive and 82–83, 90–91; questions when considering 113; time period of 129–132
coercion 44–45, 52, 60, 128; alleviation by ethics of caring approach 120; anorexia nervosa 45–47; civil commitment and 60, 105; ethical considerations 119–122; informed consent and 117; involuntary treatment 45–46; justification for 119; persuasion *versus* 46–52; power inequity and 118–119; reducing influence when treatment becomes difficult 118; threat of legal intervention 47; unilateral goals and 122
cognitive-behavioral therapy (CBT) 72, 90
cognitive disturbances 9–10
cognitive remediation therapy 90
collaboration in treatment 13, 42, 79, 81, 86–88, 93, 120–121, 123, 125
collaborative behavioral contract 86, 88
Commonwealth of Nations, civil commitment in 26

Community Outreach Partnership Program (COPP) 87–88, 90
compassion, definition of 99
compassionate use of civil commitment 52, 99–107, 129–132
competence 30–32; advanced directives and 79–84, 91, 93–94; appearance of 64; civil commitment and 41; compromised by eating disorder 63
competency hearing 30
compliance *see* treatment compliance
compulsory treatment 19, 34, 47–48, 50–51, 59–63, 68, 102–103, 105–107, 114, 129–132; *see also* civil commitment; involuntary treatment
consent 26, 30, 41, 47, 84, 92–93, 117, 125
Convention on the Rights of Persons with Disabilities (CRPD) 28–29, 31; capacity 29, 31; supportive decision making 32
COPP (Community Outreach Partnership Program) 87–88, 90
Council on Psychiatry and Law of the American Psychiatric Association 81
court-ordered outpatient treatment 23–24

dangerousness standard, for civil commitment 71; capacity criterion instead of 119; grave disability standard instead 53, 90, 131–132; incapacity to care for oneself as equivalent 36; international laws 25, 28–29; outpatient civil commitment and 52–54; overriding autonomy 114, 126; psychiatric advanced directives and 84, 92; state statutes and 22–23, 33; Supreme Court and 35–36; weight threshold and 131–132
delayed treatment 51
Diagnostic and Statistical Manual, Fifth Edition 1
dignity 28, 60, 62, 70, 107, 114, 129
distress 6, 41, 51, 67–68, 99, 105–106, 113, 118, 122
diuretic use 1, 3–4, 100
do not resuscitate (DNR) order 79
"Draft Act Governing Hospitalization of the Mentally Ill" 21–22
dungeons, patients in 20
durable powers of attorney 77, 79
duty to protect 68, 112

139

Index

eating disorders: basics of 1–13; civil commitment and 40–54; on college campuses 4; mortality rate 5, 8–9; prevalence, onset, and course 4–5; psychiatric advanced directive (PAD) 85–90; psychological complications 5–6; severe and enduring 11–13; treatment refusal 10–11
electrolyte disruption 6
emergency commitment procedures 21
emotion skills training 90
England, civil commitment in 27
equality of care 70–71
ethical considerations 33, 59–73, 119–122; autonomy 59–68, 70, 73, 119–121, 126–128; beneficence 33, 52, 60–64, 68, 70, 73, 100, 107, 112–113, 120–121; civil commitment 126–129; coercion 119–122; general ethical principles 63–73; justice 63, 68, 70–73, 100, 120, 128; nonmaleficence 33, 60, 62–64, 68, 73, 100, 107, 120–121; psychiatric advanced directive (PAD) 91–94
ethical excellence 120, 128
ethics of caring approach 120
European Union 25–28
evidence-based psychotherapy 72
executive functioning 9
exercise, excessive 1, 3–4

fasting 3–4
France, civil commitment in 25
freedom of choice 49, 104, 119; see also autonomy

gastroesophageal reflux disease 7
gastrointestinal problems 7
Germany, civil commitment in 25–26
grave disability standard, for civil commitment 13, 36, 53–54, 71; instead of dangerousness standard 53, 90, 131–132; outpatient civil commitment and 53; psychiatric advanced directives and 84; state statutes and 22–24
Gull, William 2, 111

hair growth, in starved individuals 7
health care proxy 77, 79
history of civil commitment 19–36

hope 12, 88, 115–116
humility 62, 114
Huntington's disease 90

incapacity 82, 85
incompetence 13, 31, 61, 66, 105
indifference of professionals, perceived 121
individuality 104, 121
informed consent 41, 92–93, 117
informed decision 30, 64, 126
insurance 70–72
international civil commitment 25–29
involuntary patients: differences from voluntary patients 43–45; mortality rates 45, 50
involuntary treatment 13, 19; coercion and 45–46; Convention on the Rights of Persons with Disabilities (CRPD) 28, 31; ethical considerations 59–73; informed consent and 117; outcome of 45, 59–60; psychiatric advanced directive and 83; questions to consider 61; see also civil commitment

Janet, Pierre 3
justice 63, 68, 70–73, 100, 120, 128

lanugo 7
Lasegue, Charles 2, 111
laxative use 3–4, 6, 68, 100–101
least restrictive level of care 26, 35, 54, 69–70, 115, 120, 125, 127, 132
legal capacity 29–30; psychiatric advanced directive and 82–84; see also capacity
length of commitment 129–132
living wills 77–79
lung aspiration 7

Marce, Louis-Victor 2
Maudsley Model for Treatment of Adults with Anorexia Nervosa 90
medical directive 79
medical indications, for moving to a more structured level of care 69
mortality rate: anorexia nervosa 5, 8–9, 33–34; bulimia nervosa 8; in civil commitment patients 43; eating disorders 5, 8–9; involuntary vs. voluntary patients 45, 50

Morton, Richard 1, 111
motivation to change 116

National Institute of Mental Health
(NIMH) 21
National Resource Center on Psychiatric
Advance Directives 81
need for treatment standard, for civil
commitment 21–23, 25, 40, 114
New Zealand, civil commitment in 26
nonmaleficence 33, 60, 62–64, 68, 73, 100,
107, 120–121
nonnegotiables 88, 100
Northern Ireland, civil commitment
in 27
nutrition, poor 6

O'Connor v. Donaldson 35
osteopenia 6–7
osteoporosis 7
outpatient commitment 23–24, 52–54

PAD see psychiatric advanced directive
parens patriae 21, 35–36, 126
paternalism 33, 47, 49, 52, 60–62, 68, 87,
102, 107, 112–113, 120–121, 130
patient viewpoint 44–46, 122–123
persuasion 46–52, 118
Pinel, Philippe 20
potassium, low 6
power 118–119
power of attorney 46; durable 77, 79;
proxy psychiatric advanced directive
80; treatment 80
Practice Guidelines on Eating Disorders 40
prevalence of eating disorders 4
prisons, mentally ill housed in 20
proxy decision makers 77
psychiatric advanced directive (PAD)
77–94, 123; autonomy and 87–89,
91–94, 123; capacity and 82–85,
93–94; civil commitment and 82–83,
90–91; competence 79–84, 91, 93–94;
discharge planning 85; eating disorders
and 85–90; ethical considerations
91–94; instructive 80; overridden
83–84, 91–93; overview of 79–80;
proxy 80; reasons to create 81;
revocation 84; treatment preferences
85; Ulysses clause 84–85

psychiatric hospital 20, 26
psychological complications, of eating
disorders 5–6
psychopathic hospital 21
purging 1, 3–4, 6, 53, 68, 100–101, 102

quality of life: for caregivers 105–106; focus
on 12, 78, 87–90, 100, 116, 124–126

refusal of treatment see treatment refusal
rehospitalizations 72
resentment 104, 106, 120–121
rights, balancing 41
Russell, Gerald 4, 111

Scotland, civil commitment in 27
SEED see severe and enduring eating
disorder
self-determination 26, 32, 62, 89, 91, 94,
102, 112
self-worth, negative beliefs about 5–6, 99
set-shifting, poor 9
severe and enduring anorexia nervosa
(SE-AN) 11–13, 86–90
severe and enduring eating disorder
(SEED) 11–13, 86–90, 124–126
social justice see justice
Specialist Supportive clinical
Management 90
standard of care 61, 91, 93, 113, 127
starvation 6–7, 9–10, 53, 65, 132
state statutes: on advanced directives 81;
civil commitment 22–24, 34–35, 53,
131; outpatient commitment 53, 131
stigma surrounding eating disorders
73, 118
substitute decision maker 31–32
suicide 9, 53, 69
supportive decision making 32
Supreme Court 23, 33, 35
surrogate decision maker 62

transparency 122, 129
treatment compliance: assisted outpatient
treatment (AOT) 24; persuasion
and 118
treatment refusal 10–11, 63, 100, 112;
advanced directives and 81, 84, 92–94;
anorexia nervosa and 127; autonomy
and 29, 63; civil commitment and 19,

28, 34, 40, 42–43, 47, 49, 70; by clinicians as an "ultimatum" 13; consequences of 34; overriding 28, 47, 49; validity of 93
tribunals 21
trust 32, 93, 104, 112, 121–122

ultimatums 13, 100
Ulysses clause 84–85

United Kingdom, civil commitment in 27

voluntary patients: differences from involuntary patients 43–45; mortality rates 45, 50
vomiting 1, 3–4, 7, 101

Wales, civil commitment in 27
Wulff, Mosche 3